SOURCE DIALOGUES

The Miracle Mechanism of Manifestation

GARY SPRINGFIELD
WITH SONDRA SNEED

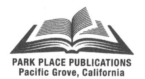

PARK PLACE PUBLICATIONS
Pacific Grove, California

Copyright © Gary Springfield, 2022

First Edition January 2022

ISBN PRINT 978-1-953120-41-0

ISBN E-BOOK 978-1-953120-47-2

Published by Park Place Publications, Pacific Grove CA

Cover design by Janet Marcroft

Interior design by Patricia Hamilton

Printed in the United States of America

To order additional copies of this book, contact:
831-224-4279 • www.garyspringfield.com

Dedication

This book is dedicated to the awakening of all humanity,
and to our exquisite Mother Earth who holds all her creatures,
big and small, within her sacred heart.

Acknowledgements

I would like to thank: My friend and spiritual brother, Ed Ferrero, for making this book possible by spending countless hours transcribing 800 pages of dialogue, and walking this path with me. My dear wife, Jennifer, for her suggestions and assistance with the design, but most of all for the extraordinary life adventure we share. My sister in light, Dew, who has always generously supported the work, assisted me in reading copy and walks the Christed path with grace. My dear friend, Marcia Kimpton, for her generous support to help publish the book, and her unwavering dedication to enlightening humanity through love, light and laughter. My brother in light, Gregory Franco for his advice and assistance with editing the copy. Patricia Hamilton, my publisher who did an outstanding job. Finally, a heartfelt thanks to Sondra Sneed who brought through this important information for the revelation of SOURCE/LOVE on Earth.

The magnificent artwork for the cover was generously donated by Anna Kumashov, sacredgeometryart@gmail.com

Prints of the artwork are available at her amazing web site. www. Cosmicarmour.com

The photo of the star tetrahedron crop circle is by Steve Alexander.

SESSIONS

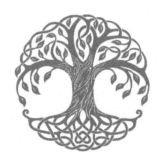

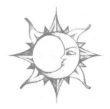

Introduction to Source Dialogues
by Gary Springfield

Over the last several millennia, what we have been <u>conditioned</u> to call God, Source, Atma, Yahweh, as well as many other names, is in fact a field of infinite consciousness that pervades the entire universe. It IS the existence of all life and matter within the universe. We are all Source/ Oneness.

The most important question we can ask ourselves is; "How did we get so far away from knowing this field of consciousness, that we already are, that so few of us realize we are?"

The answer and the solution to this compelling question is revealed through the enlightened consciousness delivering the information in this book, Source Dialogues. In order to give you, the reader, some context of a highly evolved and enlightened consciousness that has much veracity and wisdom, this intelligence refers to itself as Source (which is truth because all life is aspects of Source). As you weave your way through these Dialogues, you are gently guided by this intelligence to the revelation that you are Source oneness as well. We all made a conscious choice eons ago to explore material life for the opportunity this unique journey provided the God-Self within us to evolve. Equally important, you are at a time/place in your evolution where you are discovering that ages ago, as Source/God, you also desired to give "yourself" free will in this experiment so you could be surprised and edified at the choices you made as you expanded the possibilities of creation.

Within this expansive and, at times, convoluted journey your Higher-Self has never left you … it is the guiding light within you, the still small voice that offers signposts and clues along the way, always encouraging you to take the next step upon your path. I personally know it can be a lonely path at times as you weave your way through the conditioning, ignorance and manipulation of the power structure that has arisen in the world over the last several millennia. But with patience, commitment, and a dedicated spiritual practice, I guarantee you that the mud we sometimes slog through is a great teacher as you make your way into the light. Authentic spiritual awakening is about discovering the Higher Being or God-Self within this complex process and re-establishing a co-creative union with this Divine Self. As this connection is established more and more each day, you awaken the Divine counterpart within, and realize this is one of the most magnificent and loving journeys of awakening you could ever ask for.

The second important thing I would like to share with you is that Source Dialogues is the codex for heart-centered enlightenment. It clearly lays out authentic information about the "Christ" as the original mechanism of creation. Christ is not a person. Christ is the creative principle of the universe. *All Life* was manifested from out of the void through the Christ condition (Buddha Nature).

Last but not least, your insightful journey though these dialogues will reveal the step-by-step process for humans to evolve into the human/divine species that is being architected for our transition into a new paradigm on planet Earth. Source warns humanity, however, there is an alternate reality unraveling before our eyes; life on Earth is in jeopardy.

Quote from Source: "When 65% of the forests are gone, just like a clock, Earth knows it is time for the next cycle of evolution. Now is the time when each person must choose the future."

✵ ✵ ✵

How It All Began

In January of 2014, I received an email from my friend Ed F., describing the extraordinary counseling session he had from a woman named Sondra Sneed, and encouraging me to have a "session" with her.

On February 10, 2014, I called Sondra and without much introduction she chimed in; "Let's jump right into what Source has to say." She explained to me that she was a Source communicator. Her work wasn't channeling, that is when someone brings through another being or entity with information. She was uniquely wired so that information from an individual's Soul resonated frequencies in her mind which translated into words and/or pictures she shared.

During our session, I was amazed at the information Source shared about my Soul and my purpose on Earth. I was already dedicated one hundred percent to the awakening of the Christ light within me, but Source outlined essential new terrain as to what this actually meant and how I might accomplish it, and teach it to others

In all my years of dedicated spiritual work, I rarely found this level of Soul knowledge and clarity. Her connection to Source, which she lovingly referred to as "God talking with her," was precise and tailored specifically to my Soul purpose. Important information was revealed, not only about me, but about the restructuring of all living systems on Earth. I was deeply impacted about the revelation that life on Earth is in jeopardy ... Source disclosed that humanity must change in order to assure the future.

༄ ༄ ༄

The Work

Source outlined two main areas of the work that I was being directed to accomplish. The first one was to rectify the false and manipulative information that was propagated regarding Jesus as the "savior for our sins". His true message was usurped in the 4th century by power hungry factions in the "church". Jesus (baptized Jeshua) was/is a Christed Soul who incarnated in order to demonstrate the Christ condition to and for humanity. Christ energy is from the Origin of existence and is the mechanism of creation. This concept is fleshed out clearly and precisely in the book, along with the necessary steps to accomplish this divine transformation.

The second main purpose of the work is "the warning that is being sounded about the future". Humanity's existence is in jeopardy … but who will hear? When I first received this information in 2014, I felt uneasy and uncertain about it. Seven years later … fast forward to 2021 … science is sounding a tone of deep concern.

When I was introduced to this information in 2014 my response was, Wow! I need to do as much as I can to make a difference in the world and assure the best possible outcome for all life on this exquisite planet. I was enthused, galvanized and encouraged to act dynamically for Earth and humanity. Equally important, it was from this internal enthusiasm, excitement and dedication that I have evolved exponentially and have no fear or worry about the future. I know that Higher intelligence is always co-creating more possibilities with humanity and each individual … if they are open. If people don't hear, then pain and suffering becomes the unconscious choice.

Have no fear, live in joy, purpose your life from your heart and trust in the divine to lead you into righteousness and welfare during this great transition. Allow yourself to rest in the clear knowing that the transformation into spiritual peace, prosperity and joy is yours to have … if you are clearly listening to your inner guidance … not the ignorance and cacophony of the world. This book will help you clearly understand how your conscious, and more often, unconscious choices, create the infinite possibilities of experience.

Extensive footnotes edify and bring clarity to the information provided by Source.

— *Gary Springfield*
Carmel, California 2022

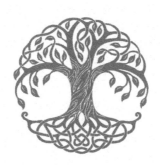

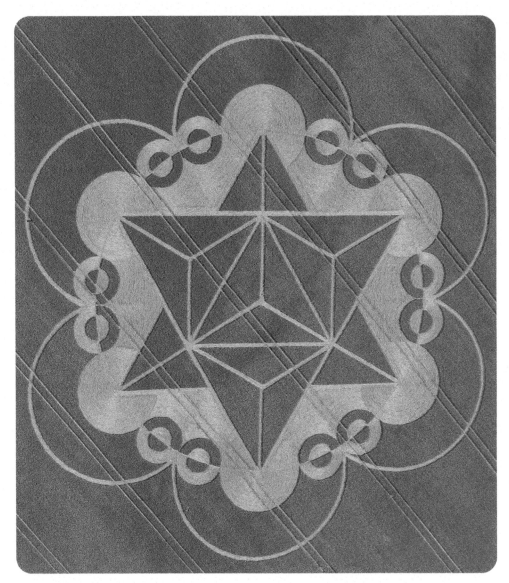

Star Tetrahedron "crop circle" created in Wilshire, England on 7/18/2017. It is 450 feet in diameter and appeared in a field where the stalks of grain were bent but not broken, as if they were trampled. (On the outer edge of the circle, on the upper left, you will notice the shadow of a human standing there.)

SESSION 1

An Important Day
2014–02–10

Gary's opening remarks: This first session began with revelations that amazed me. My Soul or Higher Self had been pre-programmed with an important "purpose" when I was still in spirit before my birth. Over the next six years I was led step-by-step into the understanding that the purpose was to reveal the Christ (or Buddha Nature) as the creative mechanism of the universe. More importantly, I was given all the tools necessary to embody this consciousness and demonstrate it in my life because Earth, and all life upon it, is in a critical time of restructuring. The solution for planetary renewal is offered in Session 4 where information about infusing Higher frequencies of light into the collective consciousness is disclosed.

The theme of disruption is interwoven throughout the book in order to prod humanity into action. Each session builds one upon the other to develop and understand the complex interweaving of forces that are in conjunction at this critical time of transformation. The commentary in the footnotes builds session-by-session as well, revealing more of the subtle nuances within some of these complex, but quite discernible topics. Like picture puzzle pieces, it all falls into place as you patiently weave your way through this loving, wise and informative tapestry of Source revelation.

SONDRA SNEED is the scribe receiving the information and each session becomes more precise, flowing and profound as she is educated by Source in the terminology of these enlightened ideas.

🪷   🪷   🪷

SOURCE: *Gary, this is the most important day of your life because you'll finally be told the things that were foretold that you would be told on this day. The reason this is the only day you're going to get this information is because from the continuing days after this particular personal invitation to your future, you will find there are people who are going to work very hard to derail you from your mission.*

The reason they are going to work very hard to derail you is because your work will have an explosive effect on some of the darkest corners of the religious world. In those dark corners you will obliterate all that is in the course of a dark field of energy. You are not going to experience this in your lifetime. It is going to be experienced after you are gone. But within this lifetime you're going to be demanding from others more than they are always capable of giving. They are always capable of giving what they believe. They rarely are capable of giving what they know.[1]

---

1   The dark energy is a reference to the First Council of Nicaea in 325 A.D. where bishops from Christendom manipulated religious documents and sacred texts in order to give the priesthood the power over the populace. They cast Jesus as a martyr figure who would save people, rather than an illuminated man who Mastered the Christ condition and showed the way for all man/woman-kind to live peace on Earth. This heresy needs to be recast in the true light of the Christ as the mechanism of creation. This was fleshed out beautifully and clearly in the fifty-plus ongoing sessions we did together. The focus of our work was to be revealed later: the techniques for embodying the Christ energy, and the gathering together of One-Hundred awakened individuals to amplify and transmit this living light into the world.

Sondra: I don't remember Source beginning a session so emphatically. Can you help me understand the essence of your work and why your Soul mission is being referred to?

Gary: The purpose of my work over the last thirty-plus years has been about embodying the Golden Light of the Christ consciousness, spiritually, mentally, emotionally, and just as importantly, physically. When we clear the emotional body, we let go of any resistance, and resistance is simply lack of love. As we are able to love the body (and ourselves) more profoundly, it opens up the possibility of restructuring DNA within the physical form so that High frequency light and consciousness can be fully integrated within form.[2]

Sondra: Wow, wow!

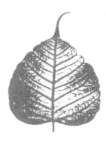

---

2   I had already been meditating with extreme dedication for 30-plus years, hosting spiritual retreats, facilitating aura readings and counseling, so I had a clear understanding of my path. But things would begin to change dramatically with this new and profound revelation in my life, which was the <u>eternal truth</u> of the Christ energy as the creative force that brings unmanifest Source/God into manifestation. The precise steps to realize this human/divine transformation was the ongoing revelation in these dialogues.

Gary: This is the mystical marriage of spirit and matter, which activates the human/divine form that already is the perfection of our Soul.

Sondra: I'm sorry Gary, I'm trying not to get overwhelmed by that.

Gary: It's pretty exciting. But it feels to me this is what all enlightened Masters were able to do. They so fully loved the body they were able to vibrate at the frequency of the Christ Consciousness (sometimes referred to as the Buddha Nature). This is the goal of evolution … to reveal the human/divine form.

Sondra: You're bringing language to this modern era. Mary Baker Eddy of Christian Science tried to do it in her time.

Gary: Correct. However, most spiritual people may know this truth, but they don't know how to clear the emotional body in order to set themselves free from conditioning and limitation. The emotional body is created from conception to seven years, when the vulnerable child is simply hypnotized into old belief systems that create emotions of fear, sadness, grief, shame, blame, frustration. These negative emotions wrap around the light body, creating lack of self-love which doesn't allow integration of truth at a feeling level. We know the truth, but until you can feel it in the body, it exists only as a mind truth.

Sondra: That's the error Christian Science talked about and what originally sin meant; *error or missed mark.* You can't be true when there is a warping that's being created by the emotional body.

Gary: That is just lack of self-love. Every emotion is made of Source energy which is a frequency or vibration; cancer is source energy, HIV is source energy, violence is source energy. It's just energy, but it is in a counter clockwise spiral of negativity. When love is re-established and we love the symbolic darkness, it (ignorance) transmutes back to become source energy once again; it becomes a transmutation of the darkness back into the gold of wisdom. Everything is source energy at its core.

If we are living, L-I-V-E, in love within the creative aspect of God; it's a clockwise spiral. When there's judgment or criticism, it becomes a counter-clockwise spiral, or live spelled backwards, which is E-V-I-L or darkness. This creates negative emotion, which is the root cause of all disease.[3]

❀ ❀ ❀

Gary's comment: Source now begins the important revelation that Earth and human existence is in jeopardy. This was a surprising turn of events for me, but Source revealed more about the problem (and the solutions) throughout the book. As each session unfolded with more wisdom and elegance one after the other, my understanding grew exponentially.

3　My work up to this point had been focused upon clearing the emotional body of trauma and disease. I realized the negative emotion we feel today was first experienced in childhood when we were vulnerable to the programming of limited parental, cultural, and societal beliefs i.e., lack of unconditional love. It was usually connected to some past life event where we caused pain and suffering to others. The negative emotion we were experiencing today was karma (what you sow, so shall you reap) from some lifetime. The people and events in this lifetime, causing our painful emotion, are simply mirroring our own past ignorance for our edification. If and when the emotion is acknowledged, felt and released we can forgive ourselves for past causation of suffering upon another. We realize that the events in this lifetime were a re-enactment of our past ignorance. The corresponding forgiveness of past events, and of people in this lifetime, translates into love for others and abiding love for ourselves ... a healing. This transformation allows the pure and perfect Golden Light of the Soul to enter into the body and be present in one's life and actions ... enlightenment.

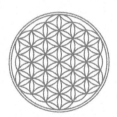

Information about the New Paradigm and this Book

SOURCE: *It's in that moment in time when dust is all there is that this is written in stone, so that those who are left can repopulate with the appropriate amount of nature knowing. It's in the nature knowing that man becomes more spirit than matter. In the nature knowing that man is more spirit than matter, there must be guiding words. These guiding words are what will tell the future humans what they are to become, so that God can be on Earth. God cannot be on Earth while All That Is, is growing from the material matter makeup of God. It is in the forest of life that man has to evolve because man is a material body. But the material body has to evolve, too. It must evolve into more forms, and in these more forms are the superior way.*[4]

---

4   When everything is "dust" is <u>symbolic</u> of the breaking down of the old paradigm that we see happening before our eyes today. "Stone" is a symbolic reference of how this information is to be saved in an indestructible way for future generations (explained in detail later). This is the first reference from Source that humanity is in jeopardy because of the destruction of resources. If humanity does implement changes, then this work will be vital information for the future seeding of a "new" human being that can embody divinity and create Source/God on Earth within themselves; i.e., living in nature knowing.

The superior way is embracing the material body in the alliance to the personality of the individuated form. Future forms require the emotional body be sustained; it is sustained by Christ consciousness. You will teach how to sustain the emotional body within the Christ consciousness. The emotional body does have a way of sustaining itself in individuation provided there is a room that is given a sacred prism.[5]

When we say prism, we don't mean the literal prism from gemology. We mean a prism in that there is a reflection of the light that is given back to the absorbing light. As it is absorbed it is reflected, as it is reflected it is absorbed. This is what will sustain the emotional body, keep it in suspension while it is identifying with a self. The self is not an archetype, the self is a Being. The Being is a knowing of its own. It is a knowing of its own when it is erecting its own nature. The own nature it must erect reflects their true nature on Earth.

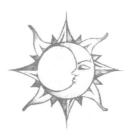

---

5   This was the first veiled reference to my true work, which would be the assembly of a "prismatic" light-form that would be constructed of consciousness and light (called the Star Tetrahedron). This energetic light-form (around enlightened individuals) is the mystical marriage of divine feminine love and authentic masculine power and assembles a crystalline energy-form that emanates the Christ light. This is depicted in pictures of Jesus when he holds his hand at his chest and there is a living light flowing radiantly from the heart. Illuminated saints in all religious and spiritual traditions are the embodiment of Source light and demonstrate the Way of enlightenment for humanity.

This is the new evolutionary form that is going to occur. In the new evolutionary form that is going to occur, individuals will begin to see light rays where they once only saw obscure light.[6]

If they can do that in the time of their body's inhabitance on Earth, God can dwell in the being that is there. In that being there is a co-creative nature that will allow God to exist in simultaneous format.

Co-Creation

Your colleague (Ed F.) must be informed more and more who he is to you. He is going to be satisfying for you, a support system that is going to help give legs to this whole thing. He's going to provide an informational trigger that is in the modern technology way. In modern technology way, systems of information need only exist for the asker to ask.

You are among those who will be asking in the metabolic changes of the light bodies in the future. When you start to eliminate all of the barriers of your own work in the way of system generation, and your colleague starts to put into place mechanisms that are working on your behalf, you'll start to see how all this system is going to play out.[7]

---

6   The awakened third eye or brow chakra is called the inner light and it evokes the light of the Soul or Higher Self within each individual. When it is awakened, an individual is able to see higher dimensional realities of light. Such an individual will no longer be looking for Source/God outside of themselves; they will be erecting their own enlightened nature from within.

7   The frequency of the physical body has to be raised to accommodate the light frequency of the Christ energy. It is accomplished through a continual inner dialogue with spirit, reflecting and mirroring the Higher Being that each person already IS. This process is centered around removing the veils of limitation that human beings are programmed into when they incarnate into physical form. As each new level of consciousness is manifested within physical form, there is a frequency shift that allows a higher level of interaction within spirit, i.e., constantly mirroring the perfect Higher Self.

This information must be stored in systems that can be re-attributed to the alignment of all that is man's making. Meaning, this making is going to be in a form that cannot be destroyed. In the form that cannot be destroyed, it will take two generations. Two generations are on their way to making indestructible forms of accessing memory. The indestructibility of this is even greater than stone.

Stone is something that human beings have learned to build upon. The ancient Egyptians built in stone not because they were of a stone age, but because they were of an age of destructing. They were destroying all that was. As they destroyed all that was, they needed to retain all that is, before all that was, was completely destroyed. So they wrote in stone. In the Egyptian model there is a way for you to understand Christ consciousness as it evolved through pyramids.[8]

---

8   Archeologists suspect there were great civilizations before the Dynastic Egyptians of 3,500 B.C., and the Sphinx can be dated to around 13,000 B.C. Science has discovered that 12,900 years ago there was a cataclysmic event called The Younger/Dryas event. It decimated life and caused great global cooling. This could explain the destruction of Atlantis and the flood myth referenced within most ancient cultures. Egyptians were saving the information from those prior Golden civilizations by "writing" in stone. Those ancient civilizations had technologies that are yet to be rediscovered today (floating large blocks of stone and precision laser cutting of granite, to name a few). This information is still hidden within the pyramid structure. In the event there is a new phase of restructuring on the planet, the information given today will be stored in indestructible systems yet to be developed. When this session was transcribed in 2014 this sounded like a far-fetched idea. But seven years later now, the Earth and humanity feel to be in trouble.

SESSION 2

Old Paradigm

The message ... the Old Paradigm is restructuring.

Gary's comments: In this session, Source does not hold back on challenging our obsolete ideas about the sustainability of life on Earth. Over the intervening years I have had many discussions with scientific and spiritually illuminated individuals who feel, as I do, that we can revitalize the unmistakable decline of Earth's habitat. Nevertheless, Source outlines the important steps that need to be implemented to assure humanities evolution. If people do not revitalize the environment with choices of sharing and harmonious action, the outcome would be untenable. One could read much negativity into this session, but solutions are always offered by Source for humanity to evolve and radically change themselves and the environment. My final footnote, along with my comments at the end of the session, offers a positive synopsis of the possibilities of renewal.

If humanity continues to trespass on Nature's rose garden, Source lays out a method to store the life-giving information in these dialogues in advanced technologies.

SOURCE: *This brand-new message is only going to be understood by those who are going to give information for the great awakening in the future. These people have not been born yet. These people have not been acquiring the information you will acquire. You are going to develop it in a way that makes it learnable. Right now it is suspended in the chaos.*

Gary, you are going to draw forth from the "unseen" an assemblage of information that is beyond the understanding of modern ways. Modern ways cannot assimilate this information because the language is inaccessible. The language that is going to be used is going to be of a technology in the future. It is not only going to be the technology of the future, but it's going to be how the technology works into the language of the future.[9]

There are ways we are impressing and programming the next stage of human evolution. When this information becomes embedded into new technology (yet to be discovered) it will be used for "universal mind" to the human mind. The embedding process of this new technology is all about also embedding meaning. When we embed meaning, what we are doing is giving feeling. The body feels meaning, the body is an impressing machine. (The knowledge must be realized and felt in the body in order to become experiential wisdom.)

---

9   The last session talked about the deterioration of the environment, and that theme is taken up here. New information which is spiritually aligned with love, light and truth, within the Christ condition, needs to be assembled for the ongoing evolution of man/woman-kind. Once the information is assembled, a new technology will store it in an indestructible format, and it will have the ability to reproduce all the subtle facets of truth therein, especially the "feeling" quality.

Humans are rapidly destroying the ecosystem and the next wave of humanity must have new information about living in Oneness as the embodiment of Source. Over the next several years, these ongoing sessions would reveal profound information about the "Christ" as the mechanism of creation. I worked with this information and embodied these abstruse concepts so it could be passed on to future generations, who must learn how to be creator-beings when technology, as we know it, may be impractical.

As we continue to develop information about Christ consciousness, what you will be doing is humanizing the meaning. As you humanize the meaning within you, your cells actually become the memory bank. That memory bank then becomes an important part of the future of dissemination of this information. Your body will become part of a system of accepting the ways of meaning through feeling.

Our problem is if humans never understand the nature of the being of God they are, they will never elevate to God on Earth, and God can never have this Earth back. If we cannot have this Earth back, then the Earth will ultimately die without us, because it cannot live or sustain life in that way. It cannot sustain life feeding on itself. It must learn how to balance its own nature, so that it begins to grow within it, and it grows within from a way of the protection of its own course. Protection of its own course is in the way of comfort. The way of comfort is in the way of peace. The way of peace is in the way of God. And God is in the way of being. All being must know itself this way, because if it doesn't, it wipes out. And we don't wish to start another planet all over again. It takes eons and eons and eons.[10]

Sondra: So, this planet is special?

SOURCE: *It's special to us, it's special to us.*

---

10   Clearly alluding to the work of creating the Christ Body for the evolution of humanity and Earth. Christ is not a person but the mystical marriage to create a light-embodied human. Later sessions would flesh out the understanding of the Christ condition as the creative mechanism of the universe. Equally important, if humanity does not evolve to co-create with Earth, the very life essence of Earth is in jeopardy. This could possibly be the way in which a species may have destroyed the ecosystem of Mars, and now it is lifeless.

Sondra: Who is us now?

SOURCE: *Us is Creator God, but it is God's aspect as related to this Earth that is its own form. If you were to draw upon the nature of God, that is the nature of the universe, we would have to be doing a reading for someone who is working in the ways of the universe. Gary is working in the ways of the Earth and the understanding of the energy Christ that goes through the Earth. That is the nature of the living Earth, the nature of the all Earth. This is who you are doing this reading for, and the reason he is a part for this, because he is one of those who was made for this.*[11]

The way this is being made again and again is through the evolutionary nature of the expression of God through beings like this. These beings, like Gary, are indeed a spring. It is a spring that comes from the Earth's core. It is the origin of all nature. It is the Being of all Christ, and the Christ nature that is the awakening of all humans who understand that within them. There are many who do, and many who will help.

It is in knowing the comfort of God that will lift and elevate humanity to the higher forms of the beings who will supplant those who are afraid. When those who are afraid are gone, and comfort is what is sustained, then all that is dwelling upon the surface of the Earth will be the surface of the being of the life of Earth.

---

11   The Christ condition is the essence of all manifestation in the universe, from the largest Galaxy to the smallest atom. The Sun is a radiant Christ field. The Earth has a living Christ field. And a human being can elevate themselves to embody the Christ consciousness and co-create _with Earth_ in the ongoing and eternal expansion of creation.

We are battling those who are wishing to make the humans into slaves all over again. We are always battling the ones who enslave the humans. It is always the nature of our ways. We come to Earth always to free the humans from slavery, and they are enslaved over and over again. This is a battle that will go on for eternity; it is never going to not be there. There are always those who stand in the course of this battle, and Gary was chosen to be among them, because that's what he wished. So long as you understand, Gary, that you are in a battlefield, you will see that the life of your course is made. The life of your course is profound; it is profoundly made. We cannot give you any more information tonight. This is only the kind of information that's going to give you a sense of mission, a sense of knowing and a sense of understanding. This is only a matter of your personal calling for it. You must always call for it, because if you don't call for it, you will stand in the way of it. [12]

What you are going to be doing in your impressioning of yourself is the mind. The mind that comes from God, the mind that is impressioning you. You will be building the mind that inhabits the body that you are. What you are going to be describing and embodying is the Christ energy, because current ways of modern thinking about the nature of the Christ is way off course, way off course.

---

12   This was my first introduction to the concept of Beings within other dimensions assisting humanity. Much information has since come forth about the possibility of an enlightened Federation that has assisted in the evolution of humanity and provides assistance for planets that are in the early stages of conscious evolution. The Federation does not interfere with planetary free will, and so some members agree to be born into the planetary matrix to play a part. I can't say that I have any personal experience, as of yet, with these dimensional beings, but I am clearly understanding the teachings around the Christ field, and the importance of the evolution of the Christ system for humanity and the planet.

The purpose of the Christ light is from the carrying of the direction of the working way. The working way is a calling forth. The calling forth is a maneuver that the internal being is doing. It is internally expressing this light in a way that calls the cells from the eternal force. The eternal force is within the ether. The ether is containing all forms of life in a form of chaos. The chaos has to be reorganized within the body, and that is done through the mind. The mind calls it forth by internally expressing the knowing. You are going to teach individuals how mechanically they do it, not just symbolically how it is done. But how the body is literally making changes to the environment it is inhabiting.[13]

Gary's comments: The reader could be dismayed at this point in the Dialogues, but I assure you, the profound offering of love, renewal and magical possibilities unfolds like a beautiful flower over the course of the book.

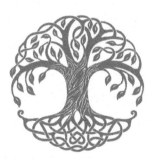

---

13 Up until now, I had thought of the "Christ" as a realized being who embodied the Divine. I was learning that Christ is a creative field of energy that summons life into manifestation from out of the void. As humanity embodies this wisdom and truth, it creates a vibration that quickens and evolves life, healing the environment as well. Up until now, all life had evolved by <u>adapting to</u> the environment, but an awakened humanity could co-create a Heaven on Earth experience.

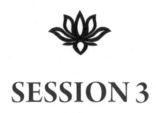

SESSION 3

Environmental Shift

SOURCE: *A creator-being understands light, and it is in the animation of light that light begins to understand what it is. Only through animation can light truly experience its own work.*[14]

Gary: It says in Sondra's book that God may lose Earth. There is actually a statement where God says, "We may lose Earth if there is not a correction."

SOURCE: *Earth is one of many, many inhabitable planets. It's just that human beings have not discovered how to find the other planets that are habitable. The reason we care so much about Earth maintaining its evolutionary path is that it's come so close to being a place where Source/God can dwell. It's getting so much closer and starting all over again just requires an enormous amount of energy. We would like to save the Earth so we can continue on this evolutionary process.*

---

14   The prismatic essence of the Christ system is what refracts, reflects and remembers light to create the holographic reality our five senses interpret as life. Through the Christ energy, light becomes materialized, which then "sees" itself in form. What we perceive as "reality" is light emanations of color so densely formulated that the five senses interpret this as manifest form. Quantum physics has shown us that an atom is 99.9999999% space, and the electron is postulated to be a fuzzy mass of thought whirling so rapidly it gives the perception of form.

It's going to take an environmental shift. Human beings have to start seeing themselves in nature, or the environment could suffer irreparable harm. If the humans don't evolve soon, they will continue to see nature as something they have to manage, something they have to control, rather than something that is a part of what they are, and therefore is the creation of what they are. Until they see that they will continue to battle nature. We desperately need man to see himself as the expression of nature before God can dwell upon the Earth.[15]

Gary: Are there beings subverting that, or is it just mankind that is subverting that?

SOURCE: *There is no real subversion of it because there is no real good understanding by even the most intelligent beings. They don't fully understand the nature of God on Earth and the importance of God on Earth. All they understand is very similar to human beings. All they understand is that there are resources that are so plentiful in the Earth, and if they tap those resources right it creates an abundance within their environmental way of living.*

What they don't know is that there is a higher level of abundance that goes even beyond that. It goes into the realm of manifesting the abundance of whatever is needed on Earth in order to fulfill any need on Earth. Evolution is constantly manifesting every need necessary. That is how there is such a diversity of life, because nature is <u>constantly manifesting</u> new forms of life, and that is the nature of the God-being.

---

15   One of the many evolutionary aspects of Earth is to produce a vessel of mineral/ biology, i.e., a physical body, and over time evolve it into conscious awareness (humans). The next evolutionary step is then predicated upon merging the human with the divine Soul and fully embodying the magnificence of the Higher Self or Divine Mind. In this way, Source or God can live within and through form, and co-create with the exalted consciousness of Earth a new and exciting evolutionary journey. Earth is a conscious being just like the sun. All orbs in the universe, even down to the atom, have some rudimentary level of consciousness, i.e., the universe is the manifestation of consciousness.

When man as an intelligent being cannot see his own God-being, then we cannot dwell on the Earth through man.

Man was created to marginalize his own ego. To marginalize it enough to create individuation of mankind, because mankind is a spirit that has no form. Each individual is the manner of an individual, but that manner comes from an ego that can easily be marginalized and thereby express the great being that is God.[16]

Gary: In my first session it talked about eliminating barriers in my system regeneration. Any specifics about that?

SOURCE: *Your systems are highly evolved; they are evolved specifically for your purpose. These systems require you to be unhinged. Whenever you experience an energy that is greater than your own knowing, it's greater than your ability to grasp, it is beyond your brain's function, you have to simply allow it to come into your frame of reference. Then you can recall it at another time when the glimpse of its particular nature is within your mind's comparison ability. It's only in the compare and contrast that the mind actually absorbs what is being taught.*

Your systems must unhinge because you are going to be taking in an influx of unintelligible information. This influx requires you to rebel against the world's telling you what your limits are. The world is making this being that is Gary Springfield into a recognizable human. They don't know how much you are not

---

16   From out of the void, Source manifested creation through the Christ system. When this knowing is embodied, and limited humans marginalize their ego, their Christed nature will summon all things possible into manifestation. No longer would there be food or resource shortages when human/divine beings walk the Earth. The process of enlightenment is not about denying the ego. The ego is as a tool created to understand and comprehend the three-dimensional world of physicality. When all that information is lovingly integrated into realization with the Higher Self, the ego naturally surrenders into exalted love/wisdom and edifies spirit.

that. They don't know how much you are an evolutionary being. They don't know how evolutionary you are. When their limitations start to create an outline in your mind about who you are, they limit what we are allowed to do for you. This is another reason why we want to start to let go of the people who are holding you back because we need you to be unhinged from world definition.[17]

Gary: Any information about the Egyptian time frame and how it relates to my working with the Christ consciousness?

SOURCE: *This information is given only to individuals who are willing to hold it sacred and understand there is no way God would allow this kind of Egyptian technology to be known in the modern world. If we let you know a few ways the technologies were used and how they came into being, then we think that will take your mind into a completely different way of thinking that allows more information for you. So, let's begin then with the pyramids. These pyramids are a form of oscillating-organic-fertile-material vibrating.*

Sondra: How is organic material vibrating?

SOURCE: *Sound. You have pyramids that are generating organic oscillating vibration through sound. What that does, it creates an overwhelming number of conditions ripe for an entirely fertile system. Imagine sound, and what does sound do for organic life? It changes its structure in order to preserve life for the crops and making a fertile plain. They didn't make sound, they changed*

---

17 Thoughts, feelings and beliefs create reality. The programming of humanity for thousands of years has fostered limited thoughts and beliefs that are built upon manipulation and control of nature and fellow humans. We are all evolutionary beings who can unhinge our beliefs, embody the divine and become master creators of abundance, peace and joy for all life on Earth. Individual choice, or free will is our divine gift to <u>ourselves</u> to wake up … or struggle through life.

sound in that area.[18]

Gary: How does it relate to my understanding of Christ consciousness and my embodying it?

SOURCE: *When you have understood how sound is working in vibration, you will understand how Christ consciousness is manipulating matter. It's in these wave patterns that are adjusted that you can start to imagine how Christ energy works through the crown chakra. What you are going to imagine is energy flowing through the body, just as energy moved across the pyramids.*

There is a direction of force. The direction of force comes from the Source of All Being and is guided and directed through the body's consciousness, just as the pyramids guided and directed sound waves to create a restructuring of organic material.

Most importantly, the feeling part is what you're going to be directing. You're going to take the knowing that you know, pull it through your body's feeling, and identify what you are feeling. It's when you identify what you are feeling that you'll be able to teach your students. There will be a significant rising in the emanation of light that has a huge effect on everyone in the room. Not only will they feel it, sense it, but some will see it, some will hear it and

---

18   The first emanation in the universe was sound (OM) that created light; in the Bible it states, "In the beginning was the word." The science of sound creating form is called cymatics and Google has many examples. The precise angles and facets of the pyramids, as well as a precise alignment with the Earth grid and star constellations, were able to alter sound waves to enhance life force and create a fertile environment. Inside the pyramid there were resonance chambers that were used to enliven consciousness as well. It's speculated that advanced sound technologies were used to levitate matter, even before the Egyptians, but the Younger Dryas event 12,900 years ago apparently wiped those civilizations out.

some will evolve physically.[19]

Gary: Anything about this great being that we call our physical sun?

SOURCE: *This is a powerful being. The only reason human beings don't grasp the full potential of the sun is because they are unaware of the tremendous nature of a body in space that is fully all its own, meaning it is contained of nothing but its own. That's a very difficult thing for humans to comprehend. They only tend to comprehend that which has an opposite, that which has a not … that which is and is not. The sun is "All Is." There is no Not about the sun.*[20]

That is the truth also about light, in the nature of God light; there is no Not in that All Light. When human beings start to imagine being within All Light and being within All Dark, when there is an imagined possibility of this, they will have evolved to a level of protection in the realm of God like never before. When there is an acceptance that All Being has of making you, the Being that can make you can also unmake you just by retracting its energy toward you. The awareness that you are making that energy come to you rather than it coming at you because of its own agenda, but that you are <u>drawing</u> that energy to you. Once human beings imagine that knowing, they become extremely powerful.

There are powerful individuals who know this entire system of drawing to you that which you wish for, that which you create. Those who know that is God

---

19   This didn't make much sense to me at the time, but it was later revealed that the focusing of consciousness and feeling can create energy wave-forms around and within the body. These prismatic, light geometries around the body open an energy vortex into spirit. This is the Christ system that prepares an individual to manifest and create reality, not by manipulating matter but by altering the frequencies and patterns that create form. It is my joy now to teach some of these techniques, which will be fully revealed as the dialogues interweave into later sessions.

20   The sun is a gigantic, radiant Christed system that has exuded out of itself the grandeur of our solar system. Through its magnificent solar life, It is purposing each planet and the evolutionary fields of consciousness therein. This is part of the ever-expanding expression of Source Oneness through the cosmos.

and love and kindness are protected by God and love and kindness. Those who don't recognize the God, love and kindness within the beingness that can be drawn and utilized are utilizing dark forces against the light. The power of the light must be constantly drawn to those who understand it and are willing to give up the dark for the pure light. That being said, we want you to understand that the dark forces that are also working are embraced by God just as you described earlier in our first Source conversation. Embraced and absorbed by God.

You described how you managed dark forces on Earth. If you can teach others that skill, then there will be a great amount of healing done that can be cascaded out into those who, as they raise their awareness, become more knowing and therefore more able to embrace all of it, and absorb it the way you have said. The reason we think you've brought the sun up in this dialogue is that it fits perfectly with your abilities to absorb the dark and make it whole again. The sun does that; it can wipe away anything in its path simply by absorbing it and turning it into its own. You are the sun.[21]

Gary: In one of the sessions, it said within my core is a wellspring of infinite Christ energy to quicken myself and all of life. Is it just drawing that force from out of the chaos and imagining and feeling it moving through?

---

21   A great teaching in that God's light is the light of the All; from out of the void spirit and consciousness emerged as light. You can summon and draw the light to you by your focused attention and feeling, and literally create your reality. This is the beginning awareness of the Christed system; the focusing of attention and imagination creates reality. Or in contrast, you can play with darkness and manifest suffering.

In the first Source Dialogue, I talked about how darkness is a counter-clockwise spiral, or "live" spelled backwards … E-V-I-L. When we embrace the darkness without judgment and bring unconditional love, it causes the dark spiral to come back into a clockwise pattern of L-I-V-E within Source Oneness. In order to accomplish this, someone has to have learned how to embrace their own darkness first (negative emotion and childhood wounds) and, thereby, love and forgive themselves at a core level which re-establishes the healing light within that is unconditionally shared with all life.

SOURCE: *The field of energy from which you draw your strength is an endless supply. This field is fed by a spring, a spring of energy that is forever and ever and ever. Most people have no clue about that spring even though they are "sitting" right on it. Your spring is over the alarm of others. When your spring is over the alarm of others, people will come to you wondering how it is you can remain so calm and having such courage in that calm. That's why they are drawn to you and why they will continue to come to you. It is all about the work that you'll be doing with regard to assembling the information about Christ energy, how to call it forth within the body, how to generate the …..(Sondra was unable to discern the word here, but it was later revealed as the Eoma. The focus of Session 5 is about revealing all the subtle aspects of the Eoma).*

But it's in this expression of your knowing that you will discover the great sensitivity required to embody the Christ. You will also be doing work related to what you're doing now, and improving it based on the information you are learning in your Christ energy work. You are constantly being fed by this spring.[22]

❦ ❦ ❦

Focusing Energy

We would like to give you a way to focus energy. Begin with the mind of your middle mind, the mind of the third eye, the center brain. It's in this place that we will formulate an experience for you. In this experience there is a work, a work of art, a work of art by your own brain.

---

22   The precise focusing of attention and feeling began to refine my body and allowed the silent mind to become more of the instrument for the Higher Self. Over time, the sacred doorway within the heart began to open into the eternal spring of Source Oneness; the field of Spring from which all creation arises forth.

Your brain has been building this structure for a long time. Your brain has been working it and working it, wanting the expression of it, wanting to know something very important. It's in this wondering that you have created a magnificent structure; it is like a crystal palace.

In the chapel of your mind there is a working of a glass crystal palace. When you begin to understand that within that palace is the enormity of you, you will start to celebrate the correction that you'll be making.

In your next meditation, in your private connection with us, you are going to begin your imagination within the center of that glass crystal palace. From there you will draw the energy that will give you the information, because it will resonate through the palace. Once you get in your mind the position of looking out from the palace and knowing everything you emanate is being reflected back, reflected out, and refracted around, it is absorbing itself as it is reflecting itself, as it is mirroring itself as it is absorbing itself. Like the sun, it will become its own being of its own way. Nothing other than what it is.[23]

---

23   This information and the exercise were setting the stage for understanding that the Christ energy hovers within the void where all possibilities exist within the mind of God. The focusing of Christ light (third eye) illuminates individual thought/images within the unmanifest, and the prismatic lens of the Christ system simultaneously precipitates it into life, i.e., everything that you emanate is being reflected back, reflected out, and refracted around. The Christ condition manifests reality in order to reflect back to God what the possibilities of God can be in its infinite potential. In the primal creation of the universe, Source posited the question "What AM I?" and there was light. The light is the Christ system that manifests reality. Christ is not a person but the creative force of revelation. This would be one of the key messages in this ongoing information and was described with ever more precision and clarity as the sessions progressed.

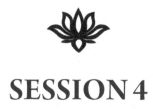

SESSION 4

The Foundation of Change

Hawaii, The Foundation

SOURCE: *We would like to start with the understanding of why you're here. The reason you are here is because the open door is beginning to close. The open door you are walking away from is the door of order in the ways of man.*

Man has an order, and in this order is a great deal of lack. The lack comes from a system that believes all abundance comes from man.

Man is not the abundance-giver; man is the abundance-taker. Man takes all that man can, in order for man to be what he wants to be, rather than what he is made to be. What he is made to be is an out-of-body Eoma. (5th dimensional light-being)

An Eoma is when the body is not the way. An Eoma is when the way is the way, and the way carries the body instead of the body attempting to make the way. The body cannot make the way. The body has no way to make the way.

❦ ❦ ❦

The body is a rock, it's just a rock, it has no instance of movement on its own. It requires the spirit of being in order for it to move in any form of animation.[24]

The Eoma is the world that exists despite the body's attempts at understanding. Meaning it is the way, the only way. The only way is the singular most important system of any system living. This Eoma is always worthy, it never questions its own nature. It never examines its own nature because all that is within it … is the examination.

If you can systematize this very order, you become more of the master. Systematizing it requires that you understand it on a level outside of the body. The body is just a tool to make it into a system that is utilized by the way of man. When man identifies what crucial elements are required to make the Eoma its own, then the orientation begins to change in the mind of the human. If you notice we change from man to human, it's because hu-man is when man and matter unite. Man is spirit. Man is individuation of spirit. Man has no gender. Man is Soul. It is also the spirit of the Soul. It is also the mortality of the Soul. It is also the way the mortality of the Soul is expressed through matter, which is the appearance of the human.[25]

---

24   The physical body (rock-mineral composition) is formulated by the Divine Mind of your Higher Self, or Soul, in order to purpose itself in three-dimensional reality. Over time, lessons of light and dark, good and bad, refine consciousness and ultimately leads to the union of authentic masculine power and divine feminine love. This is the mystical marriage that allows the light of the Soul to live fully within form and is one of the major initiations in the Christing experience. (The essence of the Eoma is further edified and explained in several of the paragraphs that follow.)

25   An important distinction is made here between human as a physical form and man/woman as a spirit that is made in the image of God and can be realized within humankind. The Christ is the way and the Eoma is the subtle substance that precipitates what the Christ illuminates into physical form. Understanding the Eoma outside the body means you have assembled the light-body of the Christ, and the glitter-like substance of the Eoma makes the light body appear as a tangible form. This is what Jesus demonstrated when he re-appeared to the disciples.

The human combines all that is mass, brings it into the Eoma, and is utilized by the Soul to create and formulate a body. The body is always at rest. Believe it or not, it is always a resting system. The only thing that makes it arrested, meaning it is a work in progress for the illuminated being; the illuminated being is man, man without a body. The illuminated being of man without a body is what the body can be when the manner of man is expressed in the nature of the Christ.

The nature of the Christ is the open way, it is the open way that transcends all matter. The Christ is the extraordinary way with which man can express man's self.[26]

The Eoma is breathing, constantly breathing. As this Eoma breathes so shall the nature of man. Man absorbs the breathing of the Eoma in order for it to assemble individuation. The Eoma is the individual nature of God, but it is also the whole nature of God.

When you pray to God you pray to the Eoma. The Eoma is the praying material. When we are being prayed to, it's because there is a reaching out, and in the reaching out is the expression within the Eoma. The Eoma is how all things are gathered in the consciousness of God. It is the flow, always flowing, always in the rhythm of the timelessness of all.

All time is a system that is organized within the Eoma. Eoma has moments of system that are incorporated because of the consciousness of the individual that wishes to draw from the Eoma into the ways of separateness. But the

26   Think of the Eoma as tiny, unseen particles; imagine one molecule of hydrogen and two molecules of oxygen, which is a gas, coalescing together to become water (H_2O) that you drink, and then lower the temperature and it is solid ice. The analogy is similar to the Eoma, but it is truly the "breathing-omnipresent" garment of God that coalesces and precipitates <u>life</u> around consciousness. Individual consciousness can "draw" into universal consciousness and build <u>the way</u> of truth, love and light. In the fulfillment of this promise, illuminated man/woman can create a light body that exists beyond physicality. They become a conscious co-creator in the ever expanding "Body of God."

separateness can never be separate, it is simply individuation from the whole, and in this individuation from the whole is a constant reflection. In this constant reflection is a creating. In the creating is a wave. The wave builds a drawing energy. The drawing energy is collected within the "One Way." As it draws to it, it creates the matter appropriate to the individual way.[27]

The individual way is a wondrous and most alarming construction. It takes a great deal of effort for it to work. The effort is coming from the individual that wishes to know what it is. As it wishes to know what it is, it draws to it all that could be. All that could be is then reflected back, and when looked at by the enormity of the individual, it is identified as that which may be. When it is identified as that which may be, it's brought to the heart to determine whether it should be. If it fits, then it is. If it doesn't fit, then it will not, and should not, cannot, and will not.

The only way to identify the individuation that is the expression of and the expansion of the nature of the origin, the nature of the origin which you call God, the nature of that origin requires that the individual re-examine, always re-examine its individuated form. As it pulls to itself that which it might be, draws away from itself that which it won't be, it is constantly building that which it is. That which it is, is a simultaneous reward.

It rewards itself, rewards itself, and until the rewards stop, it continues to reward itself with the same ongoing system of reflection. But when that system of reflection starts to fade, then the knowing must reassemble that which it might be. It does so by gathering information of that which it is, in the name

---

27   The Eoma pervades the universe and is analogous to the Internet in that it carries information. Prayer and supplication are subtle thoughts and feelings that vibrate the Eoma. It is also the subtle substance that precipitates the Mind of God into manifestation via the Christ. Human beings have their existence within and through the Eoma, much like a fish in the ocean is made of the water that it swims within. The ocean of our "Eomic" existence is the consciousness of All That Is.

of that which it is not. So it is reflecting that nature of being, not being, being, not being. When you identify with that which is neither, you begin to evaluate yourself as that which is not a body.

When you identify that which is not a body, you incorporate only that which is not a body into the body. So the system of essence becomes your only way of attraction. Essence is the attraction of essence, and when you identify the essence that is that which you may be, that which you will be, that which you should be, that which works for you to be, you begin to understand why so many are not. Why they are not, nor can be, nor will be, nor should be, because if the assembly of the nature of God begins to corrupt from the nature of man's essence, then mortal man loses direction. When mortal man loses direction there is no sense of being, and all that which is knowing, is unknown.[28]

Sondra: Is that where we are now in the nature of humanity?

SOURCE: *That's why you have to save this information for the evolution of mankind. Mankind has lost his way, he has lost his purpose, he has lost his essence. In the losing of that essence, it is a stigma. It is a stigma that becomes disease. In the stigma that becomes disease is a destruction of mankind all together. This is not what we fear, this is something that is happening. It is happening, we don't have to fear it, we are watching it. In this must be the correction, and all the information being gathered now is for the creation of new man. This began at the time of the man called Jesus. This began at the time*

---

28   The Soul incarnates to gather and refine consciousness by reflecting off of the choices that are made. Over time, the choices that cause pain, suffering and victimhood are adjusted and released, which opens the Great Way of knowing you are part and parcel of Source/God. Your essence becomes the way of love and truth, awakening the divine essence of your Soul that builds the new light body of the Christ. When humanity cannot identify within themselves the true God-being they are, they lose their way.

when he assembled the knowing, same thing with Buddha.[29]

In the assembling of this information is a knowing who you are, each one. This is why Sondra felt the triangle of the three individuals gathered here so strongly. There are more involved in this, but those who are present are among this system of foundation.[30]

Each and every one of you has climbed the mountain; you are at the peak, and you are looking out at the wide expanse. In the wide expanse is a nothingness that is alarming. It is alarming to the nature of God. It is alarming to the nature of mankind's mortal being. It is an alarm that is sounding on the highest peak. There are many peaks, but there are only a few that have made it this far. They are very important for the assembling of these components. There are many who have made their peak alone, unknowing they were to assemble with others. It is in the assembly that this has any mass. If individual messengers believe they are the one, this is beautiful in and of itself, but it is only the first step. It is in the orientation of many ones that make the foundational series.[31]

This is Intro-fusion; fusion meaning combining … intro within. This is the nature of the ritual so that fusion occurs in the moment of ceremony. It is infused in the body. Over time, ceremony overcomes the world's way and the ceremonial intro-fusion becomes the way of the body in the world. This is the nature of the Christ, God on Earth. That's all that Christ means, God on Earth. In the God on Earth way, all are drawn.

---

29   Buddha and Christ/Jesus incarnated to show the way of experiencing God/Source on Earth, but humanity has lost their way. Consumerism, greed, disease, and war create the ruination that is at hand.

30   The foundation of the One Hundred was established at the Hawaii retreat. Sondra Sneed represented the knowing of truth, Gary Springfield the embodiment of light and Jennifer Springfield premonition, the knowing of the future.

31   There are numerous illuminated beings who have awakened in the world at this time, and the unification of their light can create a dynamic force for change. i.e., a nuclear radiance of transformation for Earth and humanity.

꽃 꽃 꽃

Individual Purpose

Gary, you will be facilitating meditation by incorporating the way of focus in mind. You will be assisting students by giving the teachings of mind preparation. You will prepare the people so that they are not consumers, but beings. Beings who are externally supported by knowing spirit within.

Sondra's way is already being shown.

Premonition, Jennifer. You will be identifying where the future lies for those who are involved. This is going to prepare people who are in this selection for where the ways of man are in error. In the ways of error are the missed mark.

Missed mark is the original word of sin. For many other scribes, the word error is used instead of sin. You will essentially be telling people, such as in the time of the Bible, what is the way of sin. You are going to be telling people the way of error. This will not be done judgmentally. It will be done in the condition for what is the mark, what is the missed mark. When you tell people this, they will start to believe how everything they do defines who they are. This is the karmic cycle. The karmic cycle is all about what you do is what you are. Everything you do unto others is what is done unto you.[32]

Each of you will have a series of events that leads to your purpose as related to the foundation. There are exactly one hundred people in the foundation. When you reach the hundredth person in this foundation, you will get the new message, for the next step.

---

32   Rather than espousing sin as judgment and incrimination, the true concept is "missed mark." The karmic cycle is all about what you do is what you are. Everything you do unto others is what is done unto you. However, in the grander scheme, considering there is only One life in the universe, what you do unto others ... you are doing to yourself.

There are elements of truth that need to be revealed in order. That's the nature of this deepening process of infusion. The first group has their identifying way, the next has their illuminating way, the next has their origin way, and the final has their mass way. We give it the name, the First One Hundred.[33]

🪷 🪷 🪷

Gary's Questions

Gary: Is this why Source was saying I need to assemble the Christ energy from out of chaos?

SOURCE: *No, you are learning how to elevate your essence into the chaos so that you are no longer defined by the body; you are defined by the Eoma.*

The true Christ is an energy source for all; it is a freedom for all. That is what Jeshua truly stood for and what he taught. That teaching was intentionally twisted over three centuries by a tyrannical force. God was wiped out of the story of Christianity through the imperial manner which Jesus the Christ represented.

The Christ (that is not Jesus Christ but is the nature of God on Earth through the calling of the organization of all things possible) is the Christed condition that you were created from.

The whole illuminating origin of the nature of All Being is what is being <u>storied</u>*, and it's what is being stored. As it gets stored it is protected, because right now in man, man is being eaten alive, losing its power, and as it loses its power man just cycles down into chaos.*

---

33   Source is introducing the concept of one hundred individuals gathered together to create a dynamic wave of light and love that can transform consciousness, revitalize humanity, and pass this information on to future generations.

In this foundational way you are teaching the One Hundred how to emanate from the core outward. As each one of the One Hundred begins to emanate in that manner, truth can be stored. God's truth can be made into a whole system in man. When that is all stored, the information is protected, and all that gets drawn to that core information are individuals seeking their own enlightenment. They may not achieve it in one lifetime, but they will achieve it in a manner that is important to the ways of mankind. Those who are illuminated will carry the message.[34]

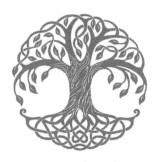

---

34   Each session, from the very first, was building upon the idea that humanity has lost its way, and new information must be embodied and then saved for humanity's evolution. When this information was first delivered seven years ago, this was new and unsettling news. As I edit this information today in 2021, I am dismayed at the ongoing ignorance and destruction of the ecosystem and each other. This information is a clarion call to wake up and re-establish peace and harmony on Earth.

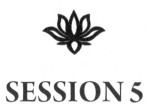

SESSION 5

Evolution of Consciousness

Gary: In the readings it was said: "The work you will be doing with regard to assembling the information about Christ energy, how to call it forth within the body, how to generate the Eoma, it's in this expression of your knowing you will discover the great sensitivity required to become the Christ."

SOURCE: *What we want you to examine first is how the Eoma is related to Christ energy. Christ energy is the way, and the Eoma is the substance. The Christ energy is a calling forth mechanism that allows you to draw into the Eoma. It is a drawing mechanism that works with the body's way of calling forth. The calling forth is a pursuing style. It pursues in the body, pursues in the way that the body experiences feeling. It's feeling for, feeling within, and feeling among the Eoma. When you call it forth, you are actually positioning yourself to draw within the great Eoma … you draw within. When you draw within it, you are pulling from the great river of Being. The river of Being, we call the Eoma, is a moving material manner. The moving material manner can be described as a system of levity.*

You are creating levity which allows you to level, alleviate, levitate, to generate these kinds of movements in the body. It is an alleviating form of moving the body.

Imagine yourself alleviating a worry. You alleviate a worry with a knowing that everything is going to become, everything is going to turn out just right. It is in that feeling of alleviation that we are describing. You are letting go of something that is holding on to you and you are holding on to it. A worry is a holding; it's holding in suspension something that causes your body to look for an answer. Once you receive the answer to your worry, you alleviate your worry ... it is a form of relaxing the muscles, it is a form of letting go of that which is holding you, and that which you are holding on to. This alleviation feeling is how you are going to generate the Christ consciousness that is the drawing forth the Eoma.[35]

Imagine a sigh of relief. In that sigh of relief is a calling. People think of a sigh of relief as a letting go, which it is; it is a letting go of a problem, but what comes in is the sensation of lightness. It's a lighter state of being. It's in this lighter state of being you draw forth the Eoma through the Christ consciousness. Christ consciousness allows for alleviation of all things that are binding the body to the Earth.

---

35   Ubiquitous throughout all time/space is the subtle substance of the Eoma. You can think of it as a magic substance that precipitates or gathers etheric particles around the images, feelings and thoughts the Christ holds in <u>focused attention</u>, and manifestation occurs. Meditation refines consciousness so that the higher frequencies of the Christ energy are infused within. Through this process, an individual is able to feel into and become One with this great river of Being called the Eoma ... the Christ is the way and the Eoma is the substance. As you draw into the Eoma and alleviate misperceptions, there is the continual enlivening and formulation of new frequencies in the body ... which are then materialized in the physical body by the Eoma as well. It is the symbolic "garment of God" that becomes your joy or your sorrow, through your choices.

The alternate condition being created here is a sense that you are rising above the body. Even though that is not what is happening, that's the sensation that will ultimately come about when you have meditated to a point of Christ energy drawing from the Eoma, because your awareness becomes part of that flow, rather than part of the assembly that is the body's material construct.[36]

The body's material construct is what's holding molecular construct into a form. The form is this body that is an individuated personality. This individuated personality is an illusion created by the mind of the individual. The mind of the individual is going to alleviate this personality from its perception. When it alleviates its personality perception, it expands. In that expansion you start to feel as if you are floating above the body. It's really just generating a wave or a frequency that extends beyond the body. In this wave frequency is a phase shift in how the individual perceives themselves. If they are perceiving themselves as a personality, and then releasing that, what gets drawn in is the alleviation of the whole birth and death cycle. Then there is a sense of foreverness, a sense of eternal, a sense of no end of the day. It is an all day, and everything ever experienced becomes a single day. This is something that heroin addicts experience and why they become addicted, because that experience is so profound the body wants to generate it all the time. It wants to know that joy. And yet, when people experience that sort of material change in the chemical make-up of the brain, it causes the body's addiction to it. If it is accomplished through the mind's manner, through meditation, the addiction is rooted in something mechanical in the body, rather than substance oriented outside the body.

---

36   Years later, in this "letting go process," I began to feel this experience of rising above the body into the fields of energy all around the body. It was challenging for the body to let go and allow the expansion "outside" the body. In later sessions, information and techniques on this process are explored more fully.

You are already doing this to a certain degree, you are already creating this. But what you are going to be doing is teaching the manner with which this is done to associate it with the nature of the early Christian's work. This is what they were doing when they were involved in the discipleship of the being called Jesus.[37]

The being called Jesus is still working on the other side helping people every single day, but the only way that personality has been able to do that is by extending beyond the personality before the body passed. So it was an easy transition to go from the body construct into the phase of the Eoma that allows for consciousness to expand into an identification with all humans who call forth the being called Jesus. This became a symbol of their personal retreat into the relationship between this being and themselves, their own being. It's similar to how Sondra is creating a relationship with us in the knowing. What you are going to do is a relationship building in the being. The being is actually more important than the knowing. The knowing is giving proof to the existence for being. Whereas the being allows for all assembly to occur. Knowing gives the idea that it's possible. Being is the possibility coming into full potential.

---

37   The One mind of Source/God individuated into Souls that were then imbued with Divine mind. This Higher mind holds the body in a molecular construct ... enclosed by ego mind, which is composed of limited societal programming and beliefs. When these limited thoughts and beliefs are resolved, the One Mind of God awakens in the revelation of the unlimited Christ within, and the entire birth and death cycle of reincarnation is negated. The Essene schools of antiquity, where Jesus studied in his early years, acknowledged and taught that "Christ energy" was a system of spiritual union. The "true teaching" is being brought to light again.

So the work that you are doing is going to have a greater effect ultimately to individuals who learn how to do what you do. Sondra is showing them how vast this potential is through their intellectual mind. The intellectual mind is the only way the body is able to allow for things that have no physical proof. The mind that is stimulated through knowing is allowed to become more aware of its own nature because of the searching that happens. The searching happens because language builds consciousness; language is consciousness. But the body is feeling; it's all feeling. It is in the feeling that when the body passes, the continuation of the feeling allows for expansion. If it is all in just the knowing, then there is a constant search for the experience.[38]

Gary: When God talks about calling, I feel that I am always calling. I wake up with the Christ in my heart, I go to sleep with the Christ in my heart. Is there a way to increase that calling, or is it more about surrendering into the Eoma and alleviating?

SOURCE: *The calling that you do now has to do with your surrender, but the calling that you're going to be doing in your deepening of your understanding is going to be a system of pulling. It's a pulling series of notions in the body. The body notes that it is pulling into itself a wave of energy that is not its own. The wave of energy that is not its own is only because it is not recognized as its own. It's recognized as something separate.*

---

38   There is an initiation called the transfiguration where Jesus is transfigured and becomes radiant in glory upon a mountain top. This is the demonstration of the body of light that lives beyond the physical body as it withers and dies. Jesus mastered the Christ system and ascended into the phase shift of the Eoma where consciousness is everywhere present. In the ascension process, the mind can know and understand these concepts, but it must be felt and demonstrated in the body to be actualized; i.e., Jesus "showed the way."

Matthew 17; Jesus took with him Peter, James and John the brother of James, and led them up a high mountain by themselves. 2 There he was transfigured before them. His face shone like the sun, and his clothes became as white as the light.

And that's on purpose, because if you floated around the world in your state of acknowledging the Eoma all the time, you would never be an individual body. You would always be floating in a manner of correspondence with all that is in the ether. Correspondence with all that is in the ether doesn't allow you to entertain the material interaction required through the senses.

When you surrender to the Christ every day, what you are doing is saying: "Take me, I am yours, and fill me with your being, take me with your knowing, take me with your surprises, take me with your illumination." But the calling is going to be: "I take you into my being and increase my being, knowing through the being you are. In the being that you are, I become, and all becoming is the nature of God. All the becoming is the surrender I am. The surrender I am is calling forth more of you within me." You do this over and over again until it fills up every inch of your body and it begins to run over. As it runs over, it is actually expanding you, expanding you. In your meditation, you deepen, deepen, and you have felt all of the great depths of the Being that you are. Now you are going to learn how to expand into the depths of your being and unscroll or unravel the original systems of the body.

The origin of all being is written in your DNA. When you expand your awareness you literally see the evolution of time it has taken to build that which you call all life on Earth. You have a moment of knowing all time exists simultaneously. When you experience that you expand to that knowing.

This is something that's going to take a little bit of time to assemble in your full being because it is not an awareness you can have without triggering the part of your brain designed for that awareness. This is where psychoactive drugs come in handy because they make it a fast experience because of what they cause in the brain to shut down. In the parts of the brain that shut down, what's left up is this mechanism in the brain. In meditation, and calling forth the Eoma, this ultimately is what is going to be activated. Every cell in your body begins to call for it. It is less like a prayer and more like an opening. Every cell begins to open to it, and when you get there, it's as if you were there all along. It's not like you are going to discover something and then it's lost. It's going to be a discovery that you realize was there all along, and you only had to turn your attention to it. It's been buried over the eons of your lifetimes, and you're finally in a lifetime where you've reached the door to knock on. It takes many, many doors to go through to get to this door. You have lived many, many lifetimes that have buried this door since your beginning.[39]

Gary: In one of our sessions it was said: "I will draw from chaos an assemblage of information." Is the chaos different than the Eoma?

SOURCE: *The Eoma is the energy flow that creates the collection of mass order from out of chaos. The assembly of chaos is done through the Eoma. You will draw from the chaos an assembly of information about the nature of evolution.*[40]

---

[39]   If you simply floated around within the Eoma, you would never master the Christ system of manifesting reality because you have to assemble the feeling in the body. If you read a cookbook, the information is in your mind but it doesn't translate into making a pie unless the body does it. This is why focused intention and meditation resolves limited thoughts, feelings and ideas in the body, and allows true expansion into the knowing of the Higher Self to be experienced. The frequency of the body is heightened and the true spiritual being (which has always existed) is revealed. The entire evolutionary journey is written in our DNA. Life on Earth began eons ago as one-celled amoebae, in the soup of original creation ... DNA holds that memory.

[40]   The Eoma exists throughout all time and space and is the substance of creation, the garment of God. It coalesces around what the Christ holds with intention and brings order and evolution from Chaos. For example, imagine the chaos in swirling clouds of hydrogen gas in the galaxy coalescing into radiant stars with planets and abundant life. Christ is the way and the Eoma is the substance.

Gary: There was a part that said, if there was an enemy takeover of the planet, the planet will not survive. Who is the enemy that wants to take over the planet?

SOURCE: *The planetary takeover is a system of dark beings who do not know the nature of God relative to the nature of freedom and kindness. These are individuals that are constantly erupting in areas of the planet that are suffering from worldly collapse. They remove any system of freedom from the populace by making promises to the populace until they have assembled governments. When they have assembled governments, they begin the dark work of taking over the planet. This is a constant battle between the humans that are free and the humans that are not. It is a constant battle and it is less obvious today because there are greater numbers of free humans than there are not-free. But that is only because there has been a relative calm on Earth. This calm will not last, it never does. It's in the preparation of the free that this is going to be eventually another battle, and we'll talk about this more because you are going to be deeply involved in the preparation of the generation who is going to be fighting that battle.[41]*

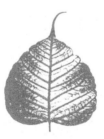

---

41   The history of our planet is steeped in war, conquest and subservience. Conflicts and wars still abound, and now there is another more nefarious aspect of manipulation and greed eating at the people, destroying resources and polluting the environment.

Gary: A session we did said, what you are going to be doing in the impressioning of yourself is the mind, the mind that comes from God, the mind that is impressioning you. You will be building the mind that inhabits the body that you are. Is this the Christ Mind?

SOURCE: *No, this is the God mind. The God mind is not the same as the Christ mind. The Christ mind is the mechanism for making the God mind. When you are making yourself the Christ, you are creating the God mind. The God mind is the combination of mind, body, soul ... it is all those things. The Christ is the energy resource for connecting those things together.*[42]

Sondra: Christ sounds like crystalline; is there a reason it sounds like crystalline?

SOURCE: *Indeed. The crystalline nature of Christ is the reflecting, refracting and remembering. It's the prism of light ... refracting the light to give it direction and reflecting the light to give it dimension. It is assembling body, mind and soul together. It is remembering what <u>it is</u>. It's like a reflection. The self, reflecting itself in the nature of the Being that is God. You are God Being ... becoming all those things.*

Gary: Some scientists call this a holographic reality.

SOURCE: *Yes, you can absolutely look at it as holographic. The hologram is just a way of creating a three-dimensional illusion. The illusion is three dimensions created from the reflection, refraction and redirection of the light. Light-encoded reality matrix is exactly the way to describe what we are trying to define through the mechanism of holographic reality.*

---

42   I was to learn several discourses later there is an electric blue field of expansive energy encompassing the body, called the Torus field. It is composed of Divine mind and is honed and refined into a jewel of living light in concert with the formulation of the Christ condition.

The crystalline nature of the Christ, refracting and reflecting light, generates the mind of God in the individual's perception of themselves. The only way to achieve God on Earth is to recognize one's self as God. That can only come in glimpses of one's imagination. It can extend beyond the glimpse when an individual is able to reach the way of the Eoma.[43]

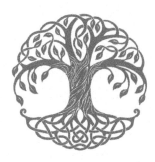

---

43   The Christ is the crystalline and prismatic field of light and consciousness that refracts, reflects and remembers. The Christ light illuminates the "Mind of God" within the void and there is reflection, a mirroring off of that thought/image. The Christ system simultaneously creates a prismatic refraction of the thought/image and the Eoma materializes substance around that held intention, and manifestation occurs.

This session began with the teaching that meditation alleviates the personality's perception of the personal ego. Over time, the awakened Christ is able to systematize the chaos in the Eoma into manifestation. Several years later I learned that the Christ is not a consciousness, but a field of energy, much like an explosive nuclear field that emanates from its radiant core. Christ is the crystalline radiance that summons from out of the infinite void all that Source/God can be in order for Source to "see" itself within form. The proficiency to accomplish this within our Earthly, mineral world allows God to walk on Earth; i.e., enlightened beings. We become realized God Beings and consummate Heaven on Earth.

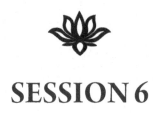

SESSION 6

Metabolic Changes

Gary: In one of our sessions, it was said that the next phase of my being is the enlightenment of my core. How do I facilitate this?

SOURCE: *You are already enlightening your core, and what you're doing is managing your life around something bigger than you. That is the One Hundred that you're starting to give yourself permission to build. In this enlightened core, is a knowing this already. You are facilitating the knowing by making the doing with each stake in the ground. You're putting a new stake in the ground every time you heighten your awareness of what's next. You are a glowing star, always walking around as a bulb of starlight.*

Now about that One Hundred list, this is not something that's going to be accomplished overnight. In fact, it may not be accomplished in this year. But it is a very special part of the work.[44]

Gary: What are the metabolic changes in the light body, and how do I facilitate that?

SOURCE: *The metabolic changes are frequency; they have to do with frequency.*

---

44   The One Hundred is the reference to the core group of individuals who are dedicated to enlivening the Christ within themselves, for humanity and for Earth's evolution.

The higher the frequency and the more often you go to higher frequency, the more the metabolic rate will change to meet those frequencies. You can't exert your forceful way without the body having its condition made either for that forceful way or against that forceful way. If it's against that forceful way, then many ailments will arise, sicknesses, not necessarily disease, but conditions that require physical interruptions to heal.

The metabolic changes will occur in balance. Every time you heighten your frequency, the body will raise its frequency to meet it. You must have periods of rest between, until such time you've built up enough of your alert way to handle the physical changes.

As you raise your metabolic condition, the body starts to work as a condition of the mind perfection rather than of the mind imperfection. The imperfections are not that someone is imperfect, there are imperfections because there are errors in thinking. When you align to a greater way, the frequency raises; the metabolic changes occur looking for vast nutrients that are plentiful, and what will happen is an ingesting of calories that will be empty calories if you don't pay attention to the type of calories that are going in. In other words, superfoods; that's a great way to see them, as superfood, because they're actually using your own super way to adjust to your metabolic changes. What you don't understand, Gary, is why. That's what we want to explain. The why has to do with the frequency adjustment your body is making. It is making adjustments to the higher mind you are penetrating.[45]

Gary: One of our sessions said that I am an evolutionary being. What does that mean?

---

45   My dedicated meditation practice, along with workshops and numerous aura readings, would move me into such a new dynamic frequency that the body sometimes went through difficult restructuring periods. (But then another frequency of light and higher awareness was enlivened within, which allowed me to penetrate to another level of the Higher Mind.)

SOURCE: *An evolutionary being is one that has made its individuation and begun its evolution and is now in a place of recognizing itself as evolving. When you recognize yourself as evolving, nothing you do can be seen as the way you are, because what you are is more than what you do. Most people are in a position where what they do is what they are, and that's their karmic cycle. What they do is what they are.*

For you, what you do is simply one foot in the world. The rest of you is evolving in spirit, simultaneous to what your body is experiencing, because you've gone past the marker, and that marker is that there is something about me that is doing this thing. You know this isn't you doing this thing. This is your being that is doing this thing, and you are observing your being doing this thing. As you become an observer to the great way of you ... knowing your being, you evolve. You are no longer going from lifetime to lifetime to expand spirit. You are currently expanding spirit as you do everything you do every day, all day long.

It's not something that has to do with how long you're alive or how much you've done in your life, or even how much you've done for spirit. What it has to do with is a Self-acknowledgement. It's a Self-acknowledgement. Gary saw something he already knew. What he saw in that knowing is himself. It was a doorway that was a two-way spirit; it was the doorway looking at its own way.[46]

---

46   As your meditation and spiritual practice deepens, you become cognizant of the Higher Being you are, and identification with ego mind falls away. It is not a denial of the ego, it is letting go of the limited perceptions that our human experience programs us with. Realizations continue to unfold until the day arises when a "symbolic layer" opens into the spiritual realms and you see/feel the Great Being you are ... and as you are looking at it, it is looking back at you. This is true Self recognition and is an opening into the Oneness where internal wisdom and guidance evolves consciousness; i.e., I AM that I AM.

Gary: Are there color and sound frequencies that we can use to stimulate healing and transformation?

SOURCE: *Yes and no. Yes, in that absolutely Source made those. No, in that most humans don't know how to do it. Most humans don't have the frequency in their own bodies to align to those colors in order for them to be helpful. They don't know how to heighten their sensitivity to those colors. We would prefer that never be brought into someone's tool chest of healing because it's a silly representation of the great way that light works. Light is profoundly significant when the light within can be balanced by the light without. But most people's light within isn't even generated; they don't even know how to turn the generator on. Without that generator on, there's no recognition of the light. Without the recognition of the light, the light can't heal.*[47]

Gary: I would like to understand so much more about light, because it is the very essence of Source Oneness.

SOURCE: **One thing we would like to start with about your knowing, with regard to light, has to do with your light and how your light stimulates other light. Your light works better than any light that somebody could fashion with electronics. Your light is an emanating power from the source of your being, and in that essence is a sparkle. That spark of light is what gives people the sudden awareness that they, too, have a light.**

---

47   When the personality is balanced, coherent and aligned there is the recognition of the Christ light, which acknowledges perfection and generates crystalline light from out of spirit/void. The purity and perfection of the Christ light dissolves all limitation with love ... and healing emerges as the true state of being. The sun is such a Christ field that generates spectacular life and light; it emanates light/love to Earth and purposes all life therein.

Even though some people will never be able to hold that light on for very long, except for when they are in your presence, it generates a fundamental change in people. You fully change the chemistry of people when they're around you. Your light projects, it doesn't just emanate, it's not just an effervescent nature, but it literally projects into space. That projection is what gives others a sense of warmth and comfort around you, because you are projecting your own being out into a room. This is what you're doing purposely, what you're doing on purpose. This is your purpose.

Your purpose is to be the being that is the illumination of those who need illuminating. You've already imagined its plentitude; now you're going to imagine its magnitude. It's ever spring.

To facilitate that magnitude, we would formulate a way for you. In the center of your being is the nature of your awareness, in the center of your being. You're going to start to bring in your awareness to that center way. Imagine yourself a sphere, this translucent sphere, and you are a red dot. Your awareness is a red dot, a small red dot in the middle of this large sphere. That red dot starts to know itself and where it is from the core of where it is, and it starts to send out pulses of light. These pulses of light are a question that says, where is my edge, how far do I go, where is the edge of me? How far does this go out? And it's in that pulsating light, that is the question of that, you will start to reverberate back from the outer membrane of your being. The membrane of that which you are. And the reason you have to reach the membrane is because your open way, meaning you don't know how far you go, where the end of your personal universe is. When it's open like that, nothing ever reflects back in the form of recognition about your power. You're going to start to recognize in your meditation an immense way that comes back, not just out, but then returns because your eminence outwardly is bouncing back from the edge of the membrane of the sphere of your being.

The purpose of this is ultimately to show you every realm of possibility in your abundant way. Everything that reflects back to you is a picture of all the realms of possibility. Then you simply turn your attention to the best possibility.[48]

Gary: What a beautiful word, membrane.

SOURCE: *Yes, it is a brain of its own.*

Gary: What is the mind of matter, and how is it manipulated to be impressed by me?

SOURCE: *The mind of matter is a mind that is replicating what you perceive. So whenever you perceive matter, you are perceiving it in your own mind. And as your mind adjusts to it, it adjusts to you. This is a kind of torrential downpour of knowing once you get that.*[49]

---

48   There is an electric blue field of energy encompassing the body. It is called the Torus field and is approximately 12 feet above and below, and 35-40 feet all around the body. It is the living essence of Divine mind. And like the internet, you can perceive and access information and higher awareness to the degree that you adjust your perceptions and beliefs to your ever expanding, imagined way.

49   Reality is the projection of innumerable wave forms or frequencies that weave and flow in, through and around you (a tapestry of light). The mind/brain perceives these, and then creates corresponding images, feelings and perceptions according to your beliefs, thoughts and ideas. When you focus your attention with clarity and purpose, then the mind of matter adjusts itself to your new knowing. In other words, it is not a static reality that we live within. If you believe that it is a static reality, then It IS! However, once you become conscious of yourself as a creator-being and know that reality adjusts to your focus and attention, it becomes a downpour of great awareness and possibilities. The Christ condition is able to accomplish this adjustment instantaneously, which is why manifestation and healing is possible for a Christ Being.

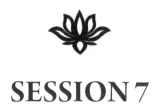

SESSION 7

Mind/Brain Connection

SOURCE: *The first thing we want to tell you is that there is a great sense of urgency that is going through you, and we want to bring that down slightly. The urgency is coming from a sense that you have a great deal to do and a great deal to accomplish in a grand amount of time. Meaning the time is grand, but it's short, and this is not true. The truth is you have an eternity to accomplish what it is you were born to accomplish. Your whole life's existence is the wavelength within which you have time to accomplish. So, don't feel as if you have to get everything that you are encouraged to get done in some limited amount of time. The reason we're telling you this is that in your sense of urgency it's also a sense of not enough. Because when you are feeling urgently compelled, "not enoughness" becomes your time, and then it starts to weave its way into everything else.*[50]

You were born in a solar system of the great and mighty force that is a system of God ... each person, an individual planet of its own. You are a "Being" within this solar system that is forever and ever and ever. There has never been a time that you have never existed. You have always existed.

---

50   The intensity and focus of my nature has always been part of my being, but I tried to relax more. The other important truth here is if you believe there is not enough time, prosperity, health, love or peace, the mind creates that to be so, because that is your belief. Change your thoughts and beliefs, and reality adjusts itself to your new perceptions.

In the realm of meditation that you will teach, people will go beyond their own sphere and into the sphere of the solar system within which they were born. As they retire into their knowing of themselves, everything they fear becomes small and insignificant. It has no meaning anymore.[51]

Gary: It is in animation that light begins to understand itself. What does that mean?

SOURCE: *Animation is the essence of life showing through that which is manifest on Earth. As things move, they reveal the life they are in their movement. When they stop moving, they are no longer the life of that movement. They are the life of spirit, but there is no proof that they are spirit.*

Spirit cannot prove to itself that it exists; it just formulates its organization. It organizes itself into some pattern so that it can at least have some organization, some knowing, even though there's no internal mechanism that allows it to see itself. When you're in spirit, you only sense the presence of others knowing that they're there; you know in your knowing the presence of the other beings.

When you're in body, animation of the body, meaning the body moves, gestures, senses, creates sensation within the body. This animation of life proves to itself that it exists. There is no sensing about it.

In spirit you are actually all in one body. The only thing that tells you this is an organized separate entity from you is the organization of the molecular system. It is organized differently. You don't see it, you don't smell it, you don't taste it, you don't touch it ... you know it, you just know there is an existence of something that is not you. And you sense Its every wave of being. You know everything about It without seeing, smelling, tasting, touching, hearing. It's

---

51   Golden light mediation is an experiential journey into the knowing and feeling of the Great Being you are that has existed forever and ever. As you rest within this transcendent experience, the worries, dramas and cares of the mundane world become insignificant.

think-speaking, so you can speak to each other through the mind. And there's the appearance of hearing because your mind is receiving what they're telling you. But it isn't really hearing, just as your thoughts aren't really hearing. But you know they're there and you can accept their knowing when you listen to your thoughts, but they are not going through your eardrum.

It's this essence of being that is in every cell of your physical body, which spirit is inhabiting. That is the animation and proof of the spirit's existence.[52]

Gary: I understand that alchemy is the lead of the unconscious into the gold of the Christ. But is it also the transmutation of material substance into physical gold?

SOURCE: *Oh, yes.*

Gary: How is that accomplished?

SOURCE: *Alchemy is just a way of describing how to manipulate the material of the elements. All elements are manipulatable, so alchemy is the construction, reconstruction, disassembly, disintegration and distillation of the element.*

Now, I think what you're asking, though, is where does the gold in the way of alchemy influence the nature of spirit. Is that what you're asking?

---

52   An interesting dissertation to understand life outside the body, whereas life in manifestation is the animation of consciousness in a cellular body to create the great illusion of separateness. In this separateness, it is animation (movement) that allows spirit to reveal Its life. Separation or individuation into physicality allows an aspect of Source/God to have free will and co-create the expansion of consciousness by choosing each new moment in revelation.

Gary: That's an interesting question, I like that question. But I was also wondering if there is an actual transmutation of physical material into gold?

SOURCE: *No. The only way to do that is through time and evolution. We do that in the system of the nature of creation, so that gold is ultimately veining through the body of the earth, because gold has properties that help bring, ultimately, organic matter to the surface of the Earth. But it has surface purpose, so it's not as if mining from the ground is going to cause any issues with the evolving nature of the Earth. It already served its purpose, and the next wave isn't using gold; it's using diamonds. Diamonds are going to be part of the next wave of the Earth's evolution.*[53]

The wave of your golden light, however, which is what we would like to talk about in relation to spirit, is very similar to how we used it in the planet, to ultimately create the organic sphere.

In the organic-sphere there is a purpose in-line, meaning the evolving way has purpose and it is aligned with the ultimate purpose which we don't reveal at this stage of human evolution. In a future state of evolution humans will know what the ultimate purpose of the evolving planet is.[54]

---

53   The concept of veins of gold interlaced through Earth really struck me, because I could see how spirit is able to move though the conductivity of gold and energize the planet and the organic realms! Also intriguing is the concept of diamonds as the next wave of Earth's evolution, because the spinning Star Tetrahedron, which is intimately associated with the Christ wave, looks like a faceted diamond as it spins and opens the sacred doorway into the void.

54   Other information I have come across spoke of humanity as the neurons, (similar to neurons in a brain) for the Great Being, called Gaia, that embodies Earth. When humanity fully evolves and awakens, we will be able to co-create with this great Being, Gaia, another stage of evolution as the symbolic and symbiotic brain of the planet.

The acknowledgement of spirit in golden light meditation, which is what you teach, has to do with creating the organic sphere within the body. That's what enables healing in the body, but more importantly the healing of spirit, because the spirit is the essence of all organic. The essence of organic is in the nature of spirit because without it organic dies. So all things on earth that are organic have spirit.[55]

Gary: In a session it was said, I will begin to cast light into a room. Is this through knowing that the higher mind, in conjunction with the heart, can imagine and create the illumination … and it is so?

SOURCE: *Yes, exactly so.*

Gary: Is the mechanism in the brain for experiencing Christ consciousness the pineal gland?

SOURCE: *Well, it's a good place to focus in the brain so that it stimulates activity there, but it doesn't come from there. It actually comes from the spinal cord. The spinal cord is what is generating all the connections for the stimulus for the brain's chemical behavior.*

Without that electricity, the chemicals just sit dormant; they don't do anything. But the spinal cord puts all of the electrical impulses to ignite the movement of chemistry.

If you want to give people another place to focus their attention, so as to enliven the pineal gland, we suggest you give them the idea that electricity is moving up their spine, and it's moving, moving up into fulfilling the needs of the brain. It's moving through the brain and then moving into the center of the brain, the apple of the brain.

---

55   Golden light is imbued with an organic frequency of spirit light within it. Focusing the light of the mind with clarity, intention and feeling upon the essence of Golden Light structures and builds organic life with balance. This is Christ consciousness. Mind is the builder and spirit is the life.

We call it an apple because there is a skin, a membrane, then there is meat, then there is core. If you think of the brain in that way, then you can imagine how the pineal gland is the core of the moment … with which you understand all things are centered within you. All things of your knowing are centered within you, the core of the apple.[56]

Have them electrify their spine by imagining light moving all through the spine. All through the spine, illuminating in a luminescence. As that moves up to the brain, electrify the skin of the brain, then electrify the meat of the brain, then electrify the core, then they will start to feel the pineal gland having some true sensation.

Gary: Source said that Gary is from a being that springs forth from the Earth's core, the origin of all nature that is Christing humans who can be Christed.

SOURCE: *Yes, yes. You are a Christing condition who is Christing more Christs.*

Gary: And by simply doing my purpose, as I do each day in my meditation, enlivening and imaging myself as that Christ Light, then the environment I'm creating in my consciousness evolves my being into that?

SOURCE: *Yes, there is nothing that you aren't doing. Everything that you are doing is in alignment with what your purpose is, and with what your imagining way allows you to do. So long as your imagining way always*

---

56   The pineal gland is the area of the third eye where the light of the Soul has an outpost of consciousness. Spiritual illumination awakens the Light of the Soul, and you can perceive yourself as infinite throughout time and space. This ability to "know-all-things" has an analogy in the internet, in that with your computer you can access information about anything. Likewise, the illuminated Soul can know the "Mind of God" in the body, perceiving unlimited consciousness; the core of the moment is within you.

imagines forward, you will always be doing what you were born to do.[57]

Gary: One last thought, I'm going to be off to Africa tomorrow. Any thoughts or things to be aware of?

SOURCE: *Yes. We want you to recognize a few things. We want you to see into the wave of spirit in that part of the world. We want you to float just above the organic-sphere and start to see how the wave of spirit works there; it's very different. And it is in the people, more so than anywhere else in the world.*

And the reason for that is the way they surrender, because they have nothing else but that. Also, what you're going to see, is the nature of survival has a completely different look in the wave of the people who do not use money as a survival manner. That's what we'd like you to pay attention to.[58]

Gary: When you identify that which is not a body, you incorporate that which is not a body into the body, so the system of essence becomes your only way of attraction.

SOURCE: *This is brilliant, brilliant, because what you're identifying is that the essence is itself a fundamental working, and when the essence works its fundamental way, it can identify itself without a body. That's what leads to the higher knowing. When it recognizes itself without a body, the body is no longer the identifier. In other words, when the body is no longer the identifier, then the essence is recognizing itself as an essence of being, so the body simply incorporates its own essence of being, and not the essence of those who would cause this being harm.*

---

57   Focused intention and clear imagination creates reality; your imagining way is the key to your evolution. The Christ system brings this into its full revelation, where manifestation and healing is an instantaneous reality.

58   The gentleness and peace I felt with the people, as well as the beauty and grace of Mother Nature, fully alive and radiant, was astounding. Money, grasping, needing and wanting seemed foreign to their natural native being. Most of humanity has lost their native way, and chaos is at hand.

Those who would cause this being harm would not have an essence that is conductive with the being that recognizes itself as being above and beyond the body that it is in.[59]

Gary: This essence must be part and parcel of the Eoma.

SOURCE: *The essence that is you is an organized conductivity, meaning, it is electrified Eoma particles, electrified into a pattern ... that pattern is the essence of you. Now that pattern is not a fixed manner. It's not fixed; it is always in a movement based on the essence of the mind, and how the mind moves and evolves. Every time the mind moves and evolves, the organized pattern adjusts. That's how the mind moves the organized patterns of the Eoma, the essence of the Eoma.*[60]

---

59   Essence is the quality inherent with the Eoma and is formulated into manifestation through the Higher Mind; i.e., the Christ Energy. When we systematize the Christ, we can occupy a physical body or exist within an etheric light-body. The ascended light-body can generate an appearance within form as a "light filled" physical construct. Jesus demonstrated this when he appeared in the "body" to the disciples after the crucifixion. An illuminated being, living beyond the body, is harmless. Moreover, when each of us purposes the higher vibrations of peace, kindness, compassion, love, prosperity and joy into our lives, we do not attract violence, pain and suffering or lack into our lives. What you sow, so shall you reap is the "Law of Attraction."

60   This is an amazing statement to fully grasp, because it clearly affirms that the Higher mind of the individual is free to work its way within the worlds of form. You can become a Master when you realize you are not the body ... you are the mind that builds. We can summon the Eoma to build the body and the life that we choose ... when we imagine and feel with clarity and intention. Simple keys to enlightenment, but sometimes difficult to put into practice when the ignorance of the world keeps calling.

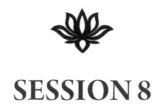

SESSION 8

Heart–Breath

Gary's comments: This session was my introduction into the <u>authentic</u> teaching of the Christ system. It was centered around "Ujjayi breathing of light and spirit through the back of the heart." With it, I felt the most amazing shift in my practice and the realization of what the Christ condition actually meant. Up until now, I had not realistically felt the subtle experience of the Eoma or the Christ system. With this meditation I began to feel a new powerful and enlivening energy flowing into the body from around the heart. Before this technique, my practice had been centered around feeling the light of the <u>Soul</u> flowing within, but this new essence was pure <u>Spirit</u>, which quickened and enlivened the body to another level. With more and more practice, I began to feel an energetic doorway open within the heart, which allowed the intro-fusion of the Christ energy into the body.

This was confirmed when I found a manuscript that said: "When love is fully established within the heart, the inner petals of the heart chakra open to reveal the jewel in the lotus. This jewel is the sacred doorway that allows entry into the void where spirit resides." At that moment, I realized this sacred jewel was the prismatic form of the Star Tetrahedron, which is an integral part of the Christ system for manifesting life.

Gary: It was said in one of our sessions that the next phase in my development was the enlightenment of my core. Is this through the enlivening of the kundalini energy at the base of the spine?

SOURCE: No, it is not the kundalini experience, it is something more enlivening. The base of the spine is for movement. It moves the body in the way of centered simplicity. Centered simplicity requires that the base of the spine be open and ready. You are going to be working in the middle of the back. The middle of the back is an area of enlightenment so profound that it is only the heart that experiences its phase shift. The heart experiences the phase shift in a way that is profoundly standard. Profound standard is what is called Ujjayi breath, Ujjayi breath in yoga. When you experience Ujjayi, you create a flow of force that creates a boundlessness, so that when you strengthen your Ujjayi breath, you become spirit. Your Soul steps aside, your body's knowing steps aside, and you become spirit.

This is where most of the information about the nature of the Christ will come from, because it is the breath that is the spiritual entry. It is the entering of the body, and when the Ujjayi breath is known by the being that is breathing, then the spiritual enlightenment phase becomes without a body ... no body at all. This is how you will understand Christ. This is how you will understand the

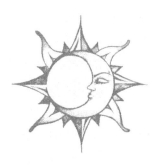

nature of perfection as it is related to the intro-fusion of the body.[61]

Gary: What crucial elements are required to make the Eoma your own?

*Source: The crucial elements that are required to make the Eoma your own is what we have just explained. It is what the nature of the Christing is. It is the entry of the Eoma into the spirit, so that the **spirit** becomes the manipulator of the Eoma. Now we don't mean you are going to be able to make something out*

---

61   This teaching was to have a most profound influence on my life. Up until now, my meditation had been focused upon seeing and feeling the Golden Light of the Soul flowing from above, down through the crown chakra at the top of the head. I would see and feel it flowing completely in and through the body and ground the light into Earth. At the same time, I would notice where the light was not flowing smoothly and realized this was a blockage. As I allowed the Golden Light to settle into this physical place of tension or discomfort, I would identify and then feel the essence of the restriction. Every blockage had a negative emotion associated with it, and as I embraced the emotion in non-resistance, I would experience a picture/feeling of some negative event in my childhood that caused me to feel unworthy and unloved. From my spiritual practice I knew this childhood event was probably related to a past life event where I acted egregiously and caused harm emotionally or physically to another person. The negative emotion I was feeling in my body today was not a random event from my childhood, it was an opportunity to understand a past life error as well. In this way, I was able to allow forgiveness for the past … and then forgive the people in my adolescence who consciously, or unconsciously, caused my unhappiness.

In order to clear the emotion, I would take some time after my meditation and feel the light of the Soul flowing into the area of negative emotion in the body. It might take a few moments, but with practice I soon identified and felt the childhood picture/trauma associated with it. With patience and non-judgment, I would begin to feel the love of the Soul enfolding the wounded child, and simultaneously see/feel the child-self letting go of the negative emotion. The picture/event of ridicule and judgment within the emotion dissolved, and I experienced a deep emotional and physical healing; "dis-ease" was released, and a greater feeling of self-love awakened within me. Over time, I was able to clear the emotional/physical body, and with each clearing, more of the Soul was being embodied.

of nothing because of your Christ access to the Eoma. What we mean is that manifesting becomes very easy; it's something that has a faster reward once you have associated these trends. It is opening the Christ into the spirit ... through the Eoma and into the Ujjayi. The Ujjayi is connected to the body; it is how the body consumes the breath, the breath of spirit, through the Ujjayi. When the Christing opens ... the Ujjayi is a calling ... it is calling for spirit. The spirit is answering the call; Christing opens up the Eoma.[62]

The reason these are two separate systems, Christing and the Eoma, is because if the Eoma were accessible to the body, it would not be a good thing for the body because the body would call upon it for too many things that have to do with physical life. The Christing is actually the conformity, it is what filters in other words, only that which is the true way for the body. Anything that is untrue cannot be surrendered to the Christ because the Christ is the true way. When we say true way, we mean there is an alignment that happens with the body and the Christ. It is an alignment with all of the cells in the body and the Christ knows what those cells are for because it is the creative force that made the body in the first place. It's the creative source that made the body and has all of the information for making a body in it. It is a tube of light. This tube is so huge that you really cannot see the edges of it. It doesn't ever appear to be a tube, but it is. It is a tube that filters the Eoma to that which is true for the body.

---

62   In an earlier reading it said, "the Eoma is the substance, and the Christ is the calling." Here is an image to help you understand this: Think of the Eoma as an infinite, small granular substance (ether) that cannot be seen or felt. The dynamic Christ system, which is the mystical marriage of divine power and divine love, holds unwavering intention (focus) and love within the Eoma and it begins to coalesce into form around the holographic image the Christ "sees." The breath of spirit simultaneously breathes life into this focused intention. It is said that the Mind of God (the unmanifest void) has all possibilities inherent within IT, and the Christ identifies each possibility and summons it into manifestation so that Source can see what Source can be. The Eoma is the substance that coalesces it into form.

The Eoma is chaos of all matter; all matter that is in some form of simplicity is in the Eoma. The Christing is the way to create the true, so that only the intention is gathered from the Eoma. Only that which is intended will go through the Christ, as the Christ calls from the Eoma what is necessary for the intention.[63]

Gary: Was the great flood created to wipe out the Egyptians?

SOURCE: *The great flood was for the everlasting nature of the Earth. It was to simplify the alignment of human to Earth. The civilization that had grown up out of the Sumerians had become far too effective and, in that effectiveness, they wiped out a great number of the resources God had put on the Earth. This Earth has been inhabited by so many other forms of life that have overtaken it, and it has been wiped out many times. The Earth is so many billions of years old in its conditional changes, and at every stage of that conditional change, there were life forms. The life forms that were in the time of the Sumerians were essentially a tribal existence and these tribes were warring all the time. In the war of obstruction and chaos came great affinity for higher forms of destruction.*

Imagine the giant dust bowls. The only thing that can follow the giant dust bowls (that come when all of the trees are wiped out, and all of the waterways are dammed up), the only thing that nature can do is blow. Because of the temperature changes in the atmosphere as a result of a great imbalance in nature, there were extreme states of cold and extreme hot. Those two extremes, when meeting, create a powerful wind and that tornadic wind draws tons and tons of atmospheric debris. The atmospheric debris moves across the land wiping out and then it settles. In the settling comes a change in the waterways.

---

63   Christ is the creative source that made the body and can only build into the body, through the substance of the Eoma, that which is true. If the ego mind could call upon the Eoma it would create a rogue representation of the true. Enlightenment is achieved when the ego aligns itself with the perfected Christ condition, which in consort with the Eoma, builds the true body.

The water ways begin to rise from the heat. The rising of the water turns into something like clouds, but it is not clouds; it is literally tsunamis in the air. This is what created the great flood. This is just the natural way that the Earth works. It has nothing to do with what God intends. God cannot stop the great floods when all of the matter of conditions are wasted. When they are wasted, the next stages that come are as dependable as a clock. It is the natural evolution of the planet. So we warn as much as we can.

This is a most peculiar matter that has occurred recently; the warnings evolving. As the warnings evolve, they start to generate great understanding. The great understanding can never change the trends. They can only change human adaptation, because the trends are too far gone, and the minds are too independent to catch on to how each individual is causing it. So many individuals keep causing it, even in light of the warnings. Those who are warning will warn others who will create adaptation. This was Noah. Among the adapters, Noah adapted to the oncoming warnings.[64]

Sondra: Was he the only one?

SOURCE: *No. He was the only one written about.*[65]

---

64   When great imbalances occur in the ecosystems of Earth, there is a disruption in the life cycles of the planet. It has occurred before, and we are at the brink of another restructuring unless we change dramatically. Also, in an earlier session, it talked about how the sun cycle was in a destructive phase and solar radiation scorched the earth. In Egypt, some of the pre-dynastic statues and temples show what looks like great heat scarring on some surfaces.

65   The first session in this book revealed the nature of this work as being a codex for future humans when civilization is in upheaval. This was somewhat difficult to grasp in 2014, even though the Mayan calendar talked about a new age beginning in 2012. In 2021 the environment, financial systems, social disruption and rampant disease are bringing the world to a point of crisis. There is a great possibility of a reset in the forces of nature because of the unabated ignorance of humans in their consumption and greed becomes more apparent. As it says in this paragraph: "There are warnings, but the masses don't hear."

Gary: How does the Sphinx in Egypt play into all of this? Was it before the flood or after the flood?

SOURCE: *It was before the flood. And it is wonderful that you asked that question.*

The great Sphinx was made as a symbol of the train. But it's not a train like when you teach (train people), nor is it a train when you are on a railroad. It is a train of sorts. It is a symbolic track.

Here is something that is very difficult for humans to understand, and it has to do with the space-time continuum. In the space-time continuum there is a traveling capability; the traveling capability is reduced to the mind's ability to see past its own physicality. This journey can take on all kinds of experiences. The Sphinx actually represents that journey. It is a journey into the knowing, the journey into the mind, the journey into the space-time continuum.[66]

Sondra: Who created it then?

SOURCE: *These were inhabitants before the Anunnaki, before the Egyptians, before the Sumerians and before the Babylonians. These were all existing civilizations that took the Sphinx on as their own. They added on to it, they prepared it, they pampered it.*[67]

Sondra: Did they worship it?

SOURCE: *Not like people worship the cross, but there was an attendance to it that was very powerful. It was used as a station of power.*

---

66   There is much information circulating today about how the enlightened Mind can fold time/space and move through the cosmos. I can fully accept this probability as my consciousness evolves and I identify less with the body and more with the Christ condition.

67   Again, much information can be found today about how Earth may have been seeded by ETs.

Sondra: Were they an advanced civilization?

SOURCE: *Oh yes, very advanced.*

Gary: Where are they now?

SOURCE: *They are long gone. And the reason they are gone is that they were wiped out. They were wiped out by the Anunnaki.*[68]

Gary: Edgar Cayce said there is a room underneath the paw of the Sphinx.

SOURCE: *Yes, there is.*

Gary: They have been doing some surreptitious digging there lately; I wonder if they are searching for it.

SOURCE: *There are too many rules and regulations in the Egyptian government for that to happen, and there will never be a time that it is opened up so long as the Egyptians own it.*

Gary: Who is the being that we call Archangel Michael?

SOURCE: *We are so happy you've asked this because any discussion of Archangels is going to give someone a more complete picture of the Soul/body connection. It is through the Archangel that this body is even possible. The Archangel is the original source derivative that created intelligence in matter. Intelligence comes from Archangels, even the higher life forms that are not earthbound but are in other sectors of the dimensional train. There are Archangels who have worked to build the intelligence and the evolving intelligence of those lifeforms as well.*[69]

---

68   Research has postulated that predating the Sumerian civilization there was an extraterrestrial group called the Anunnaki that came to Earth to mine resources for their dying planet. They used humans as slaves and may have interbred with humanity to create a biological upgrade in human DNA.

69   This is a lovely description of how Archangels were the architects of intelligence within life forms; human and even inter-dimensional beings owe their existence to these divine Ones.

Sondra: So, they are part of the original source?

SOURCE: *Yes. What they've done is individuated long before spirit became a condition for matter. Michael was a ferocious beast and his symbol, named Michael, is actually symbolically adjusted in every aspect of intelligent life forms. In other words, there are names for the Archangel Michael that are not Michael, but other names. These names can be seen in the writings from ancient times. Archangels have specific individuals who they work through in order to align the planet's intelligence.*

Sondra: How do they work through individuals?

SOURCE: *The individuals have to will it. When they will it, they become a beacon, and in that beacon their body is actually used to incorporate the intelligence quotient in one area or another. It could be in crystals, in chakra awareness, in yoga forms, in any form of spiritual acknowledgement that informs the body. Informs, in the form, informs. These are the areas that the Archangels work through, to give people understanding of the particular ways of being, the particular ways of conducting, the particular ways of inhabiting. It's an inhabitance that is conscious, conscious inhabitant. These individuals that call on Archangels are not chosen; they chose the Archangel often before they were born.*

We don't really inspire people when they are obsessed with Archangels; God doesn't have much potential with those individuals because they don't know how to acknowledge God above and beyond the Archangel. Even though they become a tool for the Archangels to inform, they cannot expand their awareness because they keep it at that form of individuation rather than into the Oneness, the wholeness of the Beingness that is God.[70]

---

70   This acknowledges individual connections to Archangels through conscious choice. But it also affirms that if the person is obsessed with this connection and they do not surrender to the Higher Being within themselves, which exists in Oneness with Source/God, they will not be "Self" actualized.

Gary: That is beautiful. When I was lecturing twenty-five years ago there was a little boy in the back of the room, maybe ten years old, and he was scribbling on paper. When he came up afterwards, he showed me the picture he had made, and standing in back of me was this thirty-foot tall being with wings, a sword and a shield. This figure looked like Archangel Michael. The young boy said he was standing behind me during the lecture. I have always felt an essence of Michael in my life.

Gary: One more question please. Is there an entity that ensouls planet Earth, a very high being?

SOURCE: *Yes, and it has its evolutionary journey. This evolutionary journey has a purpose, it has an ultimate purpose, and that ultimate purpose is to stave off any form of a no-trio.*

Sondra: The trio is like the mind, spirit, and matter?

SOURCE: *Yes. So, when you have mind, you have consciousness, when you have matter you have form, and when you have spirit you have life.*

Sondra: The ultimate purpose of the evolution of the being of the planet is to stave off, the no-trio? So it keeps producing life?

SOURCE: *Right, so that life perpetuates through the universe.*[71]

Sondra: Are there planets that have lost the trio?

SOURCE: *Yes, and these planets stopped evolving and died.*

---

71   The "Trio" of mind, matter and spirit must be maintained for a planet to survive. There is much information circulating in wisdom circles that Earth is a genetic library for many different species and life forms within the galaxy. The unique galactic "DNA" on Earth can be used to seed and terraform new planetary systems throughout the cosmos. Equally important, if human beings master and embody the Christ System, then literally God walks on Earth. There is then a transcendent, co-creative fusion of consciousness with Earth. This fusion of spirit and matter within form would allow for a new level of planetary terraforming to occur. This is why there is such a push to codify the true information about the Christ system, and to be able to store it for future generations. Evolution is going to proceed with or without humanity, but the possibilities of a co-creative fusion with a human/divine species is glorious.

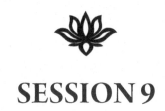

SESSION 9

Loving Self

T *he name Predator was the original title given to this session, but after going through the session to edit it, I realized that none of the information was relevant to the purpose of the book. After further reflection on the title, I realized that, in fact, I was the predator, stalking the Christ; i.e., loving the Self.*

The overall purpose of our Source dialogues, outlined from the very beginning, was defined as the embodiment of the Christ field. I was fully aware that all the information was quite profound, but it was somewhat challenging to embody and live … as I still find today! The reason this is challenging is that I am being directed by the information to create a refined light body that can hold awareness within the void and simultaneously within this three-dimensional reality. This was demonstrated when Jesus mastered the Christ field, but the religious constructs and beliefs surrounding the life of Christ have become quite distorted and limited. Humanity is now being called upon, for the hope of the continued evolution of man/woman to transform themselves and the planet through the authentic Christ field … the mechanism of creation.

This is what the statement "Heaven on Earth" truly signifies, because only through a truly enlightened human species can there be an enlightened world of co-creative fusion with/as …"God on Earth."

I thought it was fascinating how each session delved further into the understanding of how to architect the "light body". And yet, the physical body still resists consciousness living outside of its physical construct. When that scenario happened over and over in other lifetimes, the body died. At a deep cellular level, the body feels *that*; all life on the planet has a built-in survival mechanism so that fear experienced as fight or flight erupts in the cellular system. Soothing the body and gently purposing it with more love and light, along with the best environment and nutrition to continually upgrade myself, was beneficial and needed.[72]

I was fortunate that when this work began, I was living on a special plot of land not far from the sea. The air was always fresh, the grace of exuberant nature enfolded me, the sun shined warm and bright, and a loving family supported all my processes.

The awakening process enlivens the expansion of our being … but is actually centered upon unraveling previous beliefs and old conditioning that we thought were true about the world and ourselves. That conditioning is so ingrained and hard-wired in the brain and body that the process of releasing and transmuting this programming can be challenging at times.

---

72   You are not actually living outside of the body, but there is a phase shift where you know that you are present within the Torus field of Divine mind … the Higher mind (you are) that creates the molecular construct of the body in order to appear within time/space as a three dimensional being. When the Christ field is manifested and fully acknowledged, you live simultaneously in the fields of the unmanliest and manifest as a creator-being. This is where the aphorism "God on Earth" originated from.

Wisdom makes a welcome appearance when you know the challenges arise as "gifts" from spirit. Each gift awakens inner knowing that allows you to live more exuberantly and express your joy with evermore freedom when you love and forgive.

This session is about inviting each one of you to be loving and gentle with yourselves and your process. Please know that in order to awaken to the Great Being you already are ... the glory of your Higher Self ... it takes a dedication and commitment beyond belief. And yet, that is the beautiful mystery enfolded within this work ... because when you truly believe ... IT IS SO!

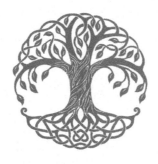

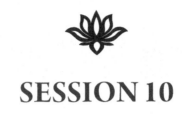

SESSION 10

Ujjayi Breath

Gary: At the beginning of our sessions source would sometimes do what "they" term a little housekeeping. This usually meant something needed to be looked at in my life and some dust and clutter needed be swept out.

SOURCE: *There are people who are working their way in your circle, and they aren't aware of the way they are working. This requires them to become really entrenched in your business when that is the last thing you want them to be. You don't want people all up in your business, because at a certain point you're going to have to retreat from the nature of management.*

The reason for that is they are in the process of learning from you how to be. You are teaching them the being of that by responding to what they learn about themselves.[73]

Gary: I've been working with the Ujjayi breathing; it is quite phenomenal. It feels like an opening within the center of my heart chakra into spirit void. It feels

---

73   Later sessions provided information about the importance of entering into pure silence and emanating light, which did open up a new teaching stream for me.

like I am breathing from the void, life and light back into this dimension. [74]

Sondra: Wow, yes!

SOURCE: *The response Sondra's having to that is, she knows exactly what you are talking about and she's feeling it as you're describing it. What that's telling us is that she is also experiencing your light when you speak. We find that incredibly important in the progress of your relationship because if Sondra understands the light within you, she will always be guided in your best interests.*

The importance of that is, as Sondra shares in the knowing of Gary's light as he experiences, expresses, and articulates it, other awakening masters will as well. The ones who are not the masters in the making will find it to be just a trivial exercise. But those who are mastering their own mastery will learn something quite profound from this blessing and it will become part of your teaching. It's not going to be just in the way of the Ujjayi breath, but also in the way of breathing in the Christ consciousness through the Ujjayi breath. That's where you're leading yourself towards, is Ujjayi Christ information, Ujjayi Christ intrenching, Ujjayi Christ consciousness.

Sondra: Through the heart light?

------

74   I originally received the technique about Ujjayi breathing through the back of the heart on 5/24/14, and this session is almost exactly one month later. As you can see, I am experiencing profound revelations about the true nature of this technique in the expression of the Christing. In meditation I began to see and feel essence arising forth from out of the void from the interior of the heart into this dimension. I had not yet discovered the mechanism of the Star Tetrahedron, (the Christ star) but that revelation would catapult me yet to an ever-higher level.

SOURCE: *Yes. The void must be purposed through the Christ consciousness, and that's what creates the wholeness that is profound.*[75]

---

75   I was revisiting this particular session for editing it into this book in July of 2021. Over the intervening years, I had been quite dedicated and disciplined in embodying this information, and I often revisited sessions and found new tidbits of information and awareness because of my continual shift in consciousness.

When I reread this section about Ujjayi breathing, an important new awareness dawned within me. As I began to feel into the meaning again, I realized that Source was being quite emphatic about Ujjayi breathing in conjunction with the Christing process. When I first began to imagine and feel spirit arising out of the void from the open doorway in the heart, I was not using the Ujjayi breath in my process. The new awareness that struck me so profoundly here was that Source was combining Ujjayi and the Christ technique as one system while I had separated them and pushed aside the breathing. The intuitional flash I had said: "You missed a vital component in this technique, so be focused with it again."

Ujjayi breathing is a yogic technique often taught in yoga classes. It is accomplished when the head is gently, but purposely, pulled back over the spinal column and chin slightly tucked in. This creates a subtle, almost imperceptible, constriction in the throat. As you focus on your breath, it is felt more along the back of the throat and slightly moving up towards the interior back of the head and the sinuses as it flows. This technique creates a subtle sound in the throat and up through the back of the sinuses as you focus on your breathing. It can produce a subtle, almost rasping, sound that you might "interiorly" feel/hear. The sound is more of a reminder that you are holding the head back over the spine and is not a sound that needs to be audible. (Although some folks in yoga get overly exuberant with the breath/sound, and I move my yoga mat to another location.)

After this epiphany, I changed my meditation to accommodate the Ujjayi technique. I would feel the head positioned a little back and over the spinal column, creating a dynamic alignment up the spine, through the head. On the deep in-breath, I focused and felt the "breath calling" spirt as the living spring from out of the open doorway in the heart. Not only was I breathing in oxygen for the body, but I was also dynamically calling spirit from out of the open doorway, in the breath. As I let the deep breath go, after holding it for a few counts after the in-breath, I experienced a subtle tingling essence within. The feeling was of spirit-breath (life) arising forth from within the void, and my awareness simultaneously experiencing the Christ wave emanating from me. The breath illuminated the Christ field, and I was the light.

Gary: So, it feels as I am breathing and moving into that place of the void, it feels like it's the home of spirit unmanifest.

SOURCE: *Yes.*

Gary: As I'm breathing it back out, it feels like it is Christ energy coming through my heart like a fountain, a torus tube of energy coming out of the heart. Then golden light begins to manifest from the interior of that place of spirit deep within the heart chakra. It's like you're breathing spirit out into this reality; that's what it feels like.

SOURCE: *Yes, yes! That is what you have to teach in addition to the Ujjayi. And here is why: people are going to experience the Ujjayi without understanding that the void relationship it is creating has a consciousness of its own. That consciousness requires direction, and only the Christ consciousness can give it that direction.[76]*

Gary: How does this relate then to the process of how the Eoma is then purposed? The void is not necessarily the Eoma, is it?

SOURCE: *The Eoma is what's drawn from when the Christ consciousness is used as a mechanism for spiritual enlivening. When the spirit is enlivened through the draw that's created from the Christ consciousness, the Eoma is the chaos of the "all" that becomes organized by intention. Intention organizes the Eoma only through Christ consciousness.[77]*

---

76   Here again, the Ujjayi is named as an explicit part of the process. The breath of spirit arising forth is imbued with conscious life and it is the Christ that gives it purpose and direction.

77   In a later session I was to learn that the void created the Eoma to be the substance the Christ system summons in co-creation with spirit in order to manifest life. The infinite mind of God within the void has all possibilities inherent therein. The Christ mechanism illuminates within the void that which should and could be manifest. Simultaneously, the Eoma precipitates substance around the thought/image and the breath of spirit gives it life ... the Christ makes it so!

Gary: In our last session we discussed how there's a tube of light around us, the tube of light that created the body. Is that part of this drawing or part of that Christing?

SOURCE: *It is the drawing, exactly. The drawing of the Christ consciousness enlivens the spirit within. The spirit within that is enlivened then takes an intention and manifests it. As that intention is manifested, the Eoma is drawn from in order to create something from nothing. This is a profound mastery that very few people will be able to accomplish in this lifetime. Only those who are destined for pure mastery are going to accomplish it. There are people you are working with right now who are in line for mastery.*

Gary: I would think that God/Source would be enlivening their consciousness without stepping over the lines of free will, while assisting in the awakening of their Soul and inviting them into this recognition.

SOURCE: *That's always the case and that never is not the case. But the truth is, it's not until they take that first step toward the light that we can actually whoosh in. For now, it's just a tinkling, like hearing a distant cymbal, like a wind chime in the distance. That's all we can be for them until they step on the path, that first step. Then we can whoosh in with a mighty wind.*

Gary: In one of our sessions, you discussed how the mind of matter is replicating what you see. Does that mean what we are visualizing and feeling in our mind is projecting out and then the mind of matter creates a holographic reflection of that?

SOURCE: *Another way of saying it that might be a little easier to grasp is, whenever the mind starts to build imagery that has profound influence, things in the universal structure start to align to that imagination. So universal structure aligns to imagination that has profound impact. Profound impact that is aligned to the way of one's purpose then becomes a self-fulfilling prophecy, and that is the true nature of manifestation. The fact that imagination is designed to fulfill purpose is the manifest of destiny. That is manifest destiny.*[78]

Gary: As I've been working with the Ujjayi breathing, in the out-breath it feels like the head region is fountaining white liquid gold through the brain that feels exquisite and yummy.

SOURCE: *It is truly the delicious experience. If you can help people understand this one thing, you will awaken in them an ability to meditate like never before. The Ujjayi is just a traditional separation between that which is managed and that which is unmanageable.*

So that which is unmanageable is the Eoma. It is not manageable in and of itself. It has to utilize the Christ consciousness in order to organize it from your intent.

The Ujjayi is a breath bridge and when you can get people to truly identify with it, then the magic of meditation will have a profound effect on their progress. It will improve their progress by many, many wanderings. In other words, their minds wander and wander, but when you provide them that tool it reduces the amount of wandering.[79]

Gary: Yeah, good word, breath bridge. The secretion that is felt within the head around the area of the pineal/pituitary gland, is that what is called amrita that begins to enliven the body at the same time?

SOURCE: *This is a word Sondra is not familiar with and so we can't give her*

---

78   Over and over again it was reiterated that imagination and dynamic focus are two of the keys to create mastery and manifest reality. When these two aspects are clearly aligned within you, then universal substance begins to architect itself in unseen ways to mirror your intention. The Christ field manifests reality effortlessly by managing the Eoma around spirit intention.

79   Again, the focus on the Ujjayi as a breath bridge. As I began to dynamically practice it in conjunction with the Christ system, I experienced a whole new enlivening in my being!

the right imagery. Will you describe it as best you understand it?

Gary: It is called the nectar of the Gods. As the pineal gland begins to enliven, it secretes another level of hormonal substance that moves through the body and quickens it to another level of transformation.

SOURCE: *Yes.*

Sondra: Is this serotonin?

SOURCE: *No. It is something completely different. There is a reuptake that occurs in the cells. The reuptake is in the synaptic region of the neurons. The neurons communicate through a gap between each node. Each node is the place where hormones are transferred. They get transferred through the neurological system when the attraction to the Source of all life is embodied … attraction embodying. To attract the Source of all life into the body is the ultimate purpose of meditation. Amrita is actually an attracting force.*

Sondra: It's a chemical process that generates attraction?

SOURCE: *Yes.*

Gary: We were discussing the sun as the Christ. Source stated there are whirls of energy at the crown chakra.

SOURCE: *By creating a tornadic experience you start to generate energy near the heart, and the heart can become stimulated into action. Eventually they're able to draw their attention away from the brain and into the heart, so that the mind is in the heart rather than in the brain.*[80]

---

80   Over time, meditation silences the ego mind and consciousness begins to rest within the heart. This is also one of the first references to the tornadic-like spin of the Star Tetrahedron around the heart, which opens an energetic doorway into the void. There is also a discipline called "Heart Math," and they have scientifically verified that the heart generates a wave of energy fifty times more potent than the brain.

Gary: Okay, mind in the heart, I like that, that's good. How can I refine myself around calling forth the Eoma, feeling among it and mastering it?

SOURCE: *Just as we described in the drawing energy of Christ energy, because the Eoma is the chaotic nature of all being. It has the source soup. In this soup is the ability to organize information to manifest in the physical manner. Everything we've described so far is going to give you a better idea how to do that.*[81]

Gary: When you talk about God with you … in the body and moving with you, isn't that what I'm seeking to do as far as bringing the fullness of my Soul, my Christ essence, and then grounding it into my body, to become the essence of God as the Christ I Am on Earth?

SOURCE: *Yes and no. Yes, that is what you are seeking to do. But no, in that it's not how you're going to accomplish it. You're not going to accomplish it by invoking it. You have to learn how to allow it, it's an allowance … very subtle nuance.*[82]

---

81   The unseen "Source soup" of the Eoma precipitates around the image/thought that the Christ illuminates within the void, and the breath of spirit brings life in order for creation to occur … from the atomic to the galactic.

82   From this description, I realized I was "wanting" this experience, but I realized the Higher Being we already are "Is" this. The enlivening process is about allowing it rather than trying to accomplish it. "Trying" is still a distorted masculine quality of manipulating to achieve. The true masculine quality of focused attention, along with the feminine principle of love, opens you like a flower to receive the perfume of spirit. Much like breathing, you simply open to receive life giving air, you don't have to try and breathe it.

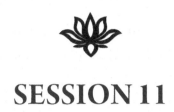

SESSION 11

RaMaNa

Gary: When I meditate there is a feeling of outrageous potential ready to burst forth from within the infinite space within the heart. Mystics refer to it as God's radiance.

Sondra: That is the brilliant void, that is what I would call it, brilliant void.

Gary: Yes, that is what it is; it is space, it's spirit, it is where "God dwells" in the unseen and unmanifest place, but it is so brimming with possibilities.

Sondra: God, what would you call it if you don't call it the brilliant void?

SOURCE: *We call it the God. That is the God.*

Gary: You're right, I know that. You can say "the God," but then in a more poignant way, people relate to brilliant void or brilliant ecstasy.

SOURCE: *Correct. What you can tell them that would be more linguistically accurate is that they are breathing in the void of creation, the void of creation. The effect is a brilliant nature within because it's only in the awareness of the great void that the brilliance of the only mind, meaning the only mind that is connected to the RaMaNa. Ra, meaning sun, Ma, meaning Mother and Na* *meaning nothingness. But it is not the nothing, it is the void.*[83]

RaMaNa. Ra is the sun, but it is also that which is light, that which is brilliance, that which is sparkly and divine. Ma meaning Mother, "that which is birthing," the ever-giving; i.e., maternal is the birthing of the giving, the great giving way. Na is the void from which it is arising.[84]

Gary: This is my feeling of what is happening; attention is being held within the lens of the Christ consciousness and on one side is the void, and on the other side is the material creation. As one is breathing through the heart chakra, one is calling from out of the void the possibilities of spirit through the heart. As it comes forth into this dimensionality, the Christ purposes God as wholeness and harmony into this dimension. Is that an accurate description?

SOURCE: *Yes. The lens creates the brilliance, that's the brilliance of the void, unmanifest on one side, brilliance on the other. Void on the inhale, brilliance on the exhale.*

Gary: As you are breathing it in, what you are breathing in is unlimited possibilities, the unmanifest consciousness of God. As it comes through the lens, "you," as the Christ, can will it into creative force that can become literally anything.

Source: Correct. It is the Christing method that allows this occurrence to

---

83   The only mind referred to here is the Mind of Source/God; the infinite field of consciousness that is called the Mind of God. This field of consciousness pervades the unmanifest void, and through the Christ system has created a mechanism to manifest itself into form. God can see what God can be; i.e., the multiverse and everything within it.

84   In these sessions Source conjures up new concepts and words frequently, and the word play of the RaMaNa with the Ra as sun, the Ma as Mother and the Na as the void was astounding to me. It summarized creation in one word and referenced the word Ra, which is from Egypt as the sun god; the Sun/Son God is the Christ ... the only begotten of the Father that manifests creation. All religions and all creation were created through the Christ system; not a person but the mechanism of purposing the void into life.

happen, because the nature of the Christ is God on Earth. You are creating God on Earth through the lens of imagination; the imagination is what turns the void into the somethingness. The somethingness is really just a reflection of the nothingness because the nothingness is the realm of the unseen; it is the realm of being no senses, the realm of existence without any proof of existence. So, the Christing manner is the way of mannering the willingness of God to be present in that which is created to be seen.[85]

Gary: With regard to our breath work, where and how does the Eoma function within this system?

SOURCE: *This question is so deep we fear we won't get to the heart of it in the training for others. We need to simplify the message, give them a picture of the Eoma in the following way. The Eoma is all possibilities, but it's all possibilities that have already been presented through the nature of the brilliance, as you might call it.*[86]

When people inhale/draw from the God, they draw into them the Source of all creation, and then, when they exhale all that is possible, they are exhaling into the Eoma. The Eoma is what conditions the environment for manifesting what it is they are true to. If they are true to their manner and ability to see, let's say, art. The Eoma is what they transmit to.

The same for things in one's environment. The condition is being set up in the individual's life if they are working towards purpose, if this is their true nature.

---

85 This description is so true and profound in its succinct synopsis of creation "from unmanifest God-mind to dimensional reality." Our imagination and intention is the lens we use for imaging-in creation!

86 I have since come to understand the Eoma as the etheric substance that the void created to give form to creation; i.e., the Source soup. In a prior footnote, I used the analogy of an infinitely small granular essence that can be summoned into density though the mechanism of the Christ field. The Christ holds power and love in a mystical union of "seeing" what Source can be, and the Eoma coalesces or precipitates the image into dimensional form.

If they are being true to this, it's becoming more and more apparent to them. Take Sarah, for example. Sarah is apparent to her diagnostic, or acupuncture way. As she becomes more true to this, she's drawing from the Eoma for it to become apparent to her.[87]

Gary: I understand that for my students, and what about for myself, though, as I am bringing forth the lens of the Christ consciousness to then purpose that through the Eoma. Where is the Eoma there?

SOURCE: *The Eoma in the Christing message is what you are going to start to imagine when you work more on the true-true. So the true-true is just what you did on Sunday. You took these teachings and you started to incorporate that into the way that you deliver information about the nature of the body's practice. Your whole life you have brought the process of God into the practice. This is the nature of your being. The process now has language because you are working with the knowing. The knowing is giving it being and language. That language is also in the Eoma, because in the Eoma is every word ever uttered. It draws to you the language that is specific to the nature of your teaching. The more specific you get to this knowing in your teaching, the more apparent it becomes to you what is the nature of the Christ, what is the Christed way, what is the Christ in every single person, what is the way they illuminate the Christ within, what is the way they experience the Christ nature they are and how is that they use this Christed nature in their everyday life. These become the specifically apparent manners as you continue down the true-true.*[88]

---

87   When an individual identifies their true calling or purpose, then conditions are set up within the Eoma to allow serendipity to work with and through them to manifest and create. If someone is scattered, then the essence of the Eoma forms into chaos and challenges for them. Most of us understand that "reality" mirrors our silent intentions and beliefs, and the Eoma is the "mattering" substance. When harnessed to the Christing, it creates abundance, love and joy.

88   I now see that this was a prophetic statement because everything that was said here about knowing and experiencing the subtleties of the Christing, has unfolded more and more each day in my life, and I know there is so much more!

Gary: In today's meditation, we took the information about breath, about breathing it in. We practiced and made it so dynamic that it began to draw to us a much deeper feeling.

SOURCE: *Yes, that is why we gave the message, "the way of purpose is coming," whether people want it or not. You are delivering the practice of purpose. Purpose cannot be avoided when you start to practice the way of God's nature within. You are giving people physical ways of practice. As they practice it, their purpose becomes more and more in line with what they do, not because they choose it, rather because it chooses them.*[89]

Gary: Yeah, that's good. Is there a specific way I can increase my brain functioning?

SOURCE: *Yes. This is within your true-true, a meaningful condition. The only reason you haven't asked that question before is because the question is completely different now that you understand what you are giving to so many.*

Sondra: Oh, that's why Gary saw the vision of the giving.[90]

SOURCE: *Right. OK, so here is the enlightened way of the brain activity for the giving that you give. The brain shuts off and what comes on is the spirit using the brain stem and spinal cord. The brain stem is what reached the outer realm from the way of the old way. The way of the old way is before matter and organic life. The way of the old way was the serpent that senses its existence, sensing, sensing its existence. As it sensed its existence, it needed to understand more of what it was, so it began to grow its brain, the processor that processes the information of that which is sensed. When you shut that off in an intelligent being, you are*

---

89   When someone gives themselves up to the path, the Great Way, then purpose calls them synchronistically to more purpose. It chooses them.

90   I had a vision that when the void opened, it became the source of infinite giving of light and life. I saw myself as a physical sun and life was pouring forth, just like a great solar being.

bringing them to the origin of all connection for God. God connected through the serpent way, which is the sensing way. God connected to God's self in the nature of the sensing way.[91]

Sondra: You mean this was before the great question? The great question of what am I?

SOURCE: *Yes. The great question of the What Am I is the sensing, sensing.*[92]

---

91   This is a fascinating description of how Source, in the beginning of existence, was seeking to know its own expression and potential. Even before light, the first impulse of creation was sound. In the cosmology of India, it is called the sound of OM and from this sound all creation arose forth. In the Bible it states: "In the beginning was the word." Sound is a wave form that looks like a wiggling snake called a sine wave. Everything in creation is a wave of energy and the size and amplitude of the wave gives it the characteristics of sound, light, heat, electricity, and so forth. When sound first arose, Source symbolically rested within this "snake-wave" form to sense what it was in its multiplicity. The sensing way gathers information at a feeling level within that which it pervades. And over time, Source was able to fashion a rudimentary brain to know what was felt and sensed. This description affirms that when you hold the thinking mind silent, you can return to the primal essence of Source and feel anything and know everything. I know and teach this because I dynamically awakened my feeling nature through many years of doing intuitive readings. I simply enfold something, a person, place or thing within my feeling nature and allow the essence embedded within it to reveal its meaning to me. I can become what I embrace without losing my identity. This is a profound aspect of love, in that you can flow into and BE what you embrace. You become one with it; in love there is no separation. This is the grandeur of sensing.

92   The void was and is a field of consciousness, but in the beginning, there was no movement within this field. The analogy would be when you are deeply asleep and not dreaming, you know not yourself or what you can be. In this primal void, Source stirred to wakefulness, and asked the question "what am I" and the movement of creation began. The Great Dreamer was now able to dream its existence in order to see what it could be. We are that dream but we are also that dreamer that created us. However, we forgot Our Self and think we are just the manifest dream. Enlightenment is waking up in the dream and realizing your innate God-being, so that you can now consciously dream the ongoing evolution of existence. This is the Christ.

Sondra: So the sensing became so phenomenal that it split the first cell?

SOURCE: *No, not exactly. The sensing was the Soul of the question.*

Sondra: Oh, so it proceeded language.

SOURCE: *Correct. This is the nature of your searching, Sondra. Whenever you search for a word, you are searching in the feeling, you're sensing and it has no dimension to it, it's just a sensing. In the sensing of that you have to call upon the things that you know, and when you can't because you don't know this thing, you sense it out in your mind. You are using the serpent way. This is the serpent way of searching the mind, searching, searching. Gary's serpent occurs when he is self-reflective, when he is looking into himself for the ways of his no-knowing. When he looks into the ways of his no-knowing he finds himself, and when he finds himself, he identifies what he must do about that. The sensing way is the nature of the no-sensation. There's nothing in you that tells you what's actually happening. You simply understand it by what is being given to you from your awareness. Then you put pictures on it, and you put language to it, and you put your identity in it. This nature of the searching is the nature of the God in the void. The nature of God in the void must breathe life into that which it is sensing. Then it becomes a material construct to reflect back to the being of God that which it is. This is why it is so important for people to be on the true path, because if they project outside of them what it is about them that isn't true, then they reflect the untrue and that reflection never gets them to who they are, and who they should be in the realm of God, which is why it is dangerous if their body passes. They are still locked in the un-true nature of seeing themselves. They can get trapped on Earth because Earth is the only program for reflection from a sensory way.*[93]

---

93   By study, reading and reflection, the mind can "know" that you are Source/God, but until you feel that, it is just a mental construct. Enlightenment is the ability to know and feel yourself as the Oneness of Source Being. It is only an embodied state of being, Earthly existence, that allows for this possibility.

Gary: Quite profound. It is the sensing way that I focus on during our retreats because we are exercising the feeling muscle. The feeling muscle and the sensing muscle are the same muscle. When you silence the thinking mind and settle into the feeling, it allows you to know anything. You could just sense it.

Gary: So, one last question. How do I use the Christ consciousness to begin to manipulate and restructure organic material?

SOURCE: *You already use it a lot more than you think you do. The ways of it are transmutable, meaning you can appoint yourself a device that triggers it so you can better understand the system. A system of understanding can be appointed so that your mind recognizes the moment you begin using it, and then can identify what the results are. You then have points in between that have been identified. The way that you are doing it now is somewhat unconscious. If you want it to be more conscious and cognizant, then it requires the mnemonic device. So let's say you decide you want to manifest a trip to tribal Africa. You would place in your mind the first notion. The first notion is to understand the reason you want to go. The second notion is to possess everything that would prepare you for the opportunity. You research it to such a level that it becomes a part of your knowing that this is going to happen. You may not have all of the hows and wherefores, but you know inside that this is going to happen, and this is going to happen soon. Then you put in the next notion the date you are projecting that you will go there. Then that date starts pulling you toward it, because you have given yourself an objective. So this is the Christing way. On an unconscious level, it works in the same way, but being conscious of it helps it work faster and more predictably.*[94]

---

94   Mnemonic devices are techniques a person can use to help them improve their ability to remember something. It's a memory technique to help your brain better encode and recall important information and, in the example above, to implement some specific idea or choice.

Gary: I assume I could use a similar approach to create more powerful, youthful and supple physical form. I would keep calling it forth, seeing it, purposing it with the Christ consciousness.

SOURCE: *Yes, and there are limits even to something of that nature, because you are working against the ways of the environment. The ways of the environment are continuously creating a drain on youthfulness, constantly. You may be using this conscious effort to ward off what's happening every day. When you want to overstep that so that it is something of great obviousness to others, (your youthful way being so obvious in the way you look and act), the way to do that is to transcend physicality.*[95]

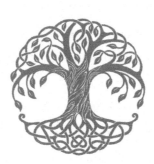

---

95   Transcending physicality means to create the light body, also known as the body of ascension, so that you can be within form or in the light body as you choose. Thus, Jesus can still appear to individuals, as he did to his disciples, because he mastered the Christ field before passing.

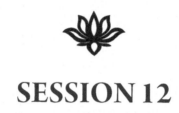

SESSION 12

Vibration of Source

Gary: Is there anything I can do to enliven and quicken my purposing of the Christ consciousness?

SOURCE: *Yes. The next thing that we will teach you, that you will be passing on to your students, is the Ah-La transcendence. Some people may worry about the use of the term Ah-La, because of its Islamic association. Ah-La is not Islamic. Ah-La goes back much, much further than Islam. Ah-La is the AH....Ahhhhhhhhhh (Sondra sounding the prolonged sound) of God. The La is the melodious nature of the symphony of life. So Ahhhhh-Laaaaaa, is the Christening of the foundation of human life, the Christening power; Ahhhh-Laaaa. The idea here is you will generate the Christening power through a chanted form of honing light.*

The first group to perform this Ah-La Christening is the group of individuals who are most interested in the Christed way. They don't have to be in the highest order of masters, they just need to be among the most interested. They have to be individuals who are not superstitious. Superstition will cause a level of doubt that creates a conflict with the power of the Ah-La. When Ah-La became the name of God in Islam, it actually destroyed the nature of the chant, because people became very uncomfortable with calling on God in a chanted form. People felt the power of it and felt it was disrespectful, so this stopped being a religious ceremony. So people will be indoctrinated with the new idea, and they are going to have to let go of their previous suspicions about it; to know this is not the name of God, it never was the name of God, it has always been the Christing manner. It's only when Jeshua brought this into the nature of Judaism that it began to usurp the former meaning.[96]

Now let's describe how you perform the Ah-La. This is a breathing and a vocalization. The vocalization is like the Om, and the breathing is like the yogic breath, (Ujjayi breathing). In the yogic breath there is a breathing that goes behind the sinuses, and behind the sinuses there is a vibration that occurs within the sinuses. It sounds this way. Ahhhhhhhhh Laaaaaaaaa <one full note higher>.[97]

Sondra: (Sondra coughed.) This is embarrassing.

SOURCE: *Don't worry, Sondra, this is going to be common, and people are going to practice it until it gets really good. When it is really good there's a vibration that occurs in the group that is enlivening. Let's try it again.*

---

96   Jesus understood the unique quality of the Ah-La as a vibrational tone connected to the Christ frequency. The priesthood bastardized it as a religious concept with a negative connotation.

97   In an earlier session, I explained how my recognition of the Ujjayi breath, as a dynamic component of the Christing, rekindled a new understanding of this important breath technique. In this passage I was struck by another important realization that there is a subtle breathing behind the sinuses. When I practiced this in my meditation, I could feel a wholeness being dynamically aligned within the body like never before. There was a greater feeling of space within the molecules for spirit to flow around and through the head/neck region. There was also a feeling of ease as I allowed my awareness to co-exist outside the body in the higher vibrational fields that circumscribe the body; Ujjayi Christ awareness, Ujjayi Christ entrenching!

Sondra: So I'm breathing in the yogic breath and I'm exhaling out while sounding the Ah-La like the Om sound as the Ah. Then same thing with the LA inhale yogic breath and while exhaling sound the La___ sounding the Ah-La three times. <In breath> Ahhhhhhhhh <In breath> Laaaaaaaaa <In breath> Ahhhhhhhhh <In breath> Laaaaaaaaa <In breath> Ahhhhhhhhh <In breath>Laaaaaaaaa.

SOURCE: *This is the beginning of it, and in this beginning there is a light-headedness that occurs. In the light-headedness there will be a silence afterward that allows the light-headedness to subside. As it subsides, there is a kinesthetic occurrence.*

This kinesthetic occurrence is then what's going to be used in the next session of it. For the next session of it is <In breath> Ahhhhhhhhh <In breath> Laaaaaaaaa. Do that three times. But when the final session is complete, there will be a relaxing into the silence. In that relaxing into the silence is an unfolding.

In the next phase there is a separation of the voices into groups followed by singing in rounds. Before this even begins, we will number people off; one, two, one, two, one, two. All of the twos will be the recall, the ones will be the call. So on the Ah tone from the ones, there will be a simultaneous La tone with the twos. Then Ah from the twos and La from the ones and so on in rounds.

Gary: How long should we do the chanting?

SOURCE: *It will be a series of three. The first three, which is session one, will get everyone's voice and their breathing in sync. Everyone's lung capacity is different. So, if you can inhale enough in three counts, then use counts of three on the exhale. Everyone will have enough inhale capacity to exhale the first three counts. Those that can go longer will make it longer. So it will be: Session one, everyone counts on the three. The exhale sound is three counts. The second session is the same.*

The third session is the separation of voices, the call and recall. Now you are going to do this at the beginning of the meditation and at the end of the meditation. This is the bulk of what we want to show you for the next teaching.[98]

After the Ah-La, you will still share the usual meditation teaching so that people understand the void and the Christ; the inhale from the void and exhale the Christ.[99]

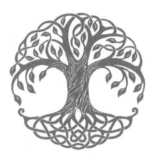

---

98   This references the musical term "singing in rounds," where individuals sing separate parts of the same refrain. When we performed the rounds of the Ah-La there was an echoing resonance which created an enlivening feeling in the body.

99   The Ujjayi breath summons and calls spirit from out of the open doorway within the heart (the interior doorway into the void). The focusing of intention and imagination within the Christ condition on the exhale unifies spirit/breath with Christ light. This is the mechanism of creation. This creates a holographic light form that the Eoma precipitates subtle substance around to create three-dimensional reality.

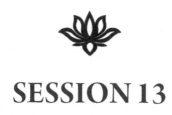

SESSION 13

Sound as Creative Power

SOURCE: *This is the training you will facilitate in the Ah-La. The Ah-La is the calling forth and the energy that surrounds the nature of you and those around you, in the Eoma taking its place.*[100]

An individual's creative power gets called upon with the Ah-La, and in that creative power is the Christing of all natures. Christing is this crackling of instantaneous knowing. The crackling of space is the Christing of all natures. When you Christ your own nature, you are taking into yourself the creative bounty and organizing it; you do that with intention. The intention is based on how you wish to create the next boundaries of your existence. All boundaries of existence are identified by experience. When the experience is of dark looming loss (negative emotions), then the Eoma can be called in to fulfill that which was lost. When trust is lost because of childhood wounds, the Eoma fills in those places that are the holes left behind. All holes left behind drain your energy.

Each experience has built the individual knowing of themselves, and in this lifetime, they know themselves based on this experience. They also draw the

---

100   The Ah-La is the vibration of the creative power of Source/God calling God into form. The Eoma taking its place means to organize the infinite possibilities of God through the creative mechanism of the Christ. It is the Eoma that precipitates thought/ images into reality; i.e., taking "its" place in physicality.

experience of previous lifetimes in order to overcome. But each wound creates holes and loss and creates hoarding in the strange ways the body attempts to fulfill what is lost. So it becomes out of balance. The out of balance is creating both loss in the structure and hoarding in the attempt to overcome. The attempt to overcome is calling upon things that are not of the great way. And when it is not of the great way, then the holes get filled with things that never fill the holes.[101]

Gary, you as teacher become a conditioner of experience because you call upon the Eoma expressing itself from within you, and as it expresses itself from within you as teacher, the student will call upon this at your call. When you start to alter their experience, then you start to alter how individuals progress in the world, because experience is how you foundationally express who you are. When you alter that because of your sense of worth that you discover through the Ah-La, you are discovering there is actually something greater than you ever imagined. This is the nature of you and your students as they are within the Ah-La.

You have expanded your being, and they are going to experience your expandedness. In the experience of that expandedness, you are going to experience your own expansion, because that is what your students are reflecting back to you. And when you see the grandness of it, and you continue to humble

---

101   I have facilitated hundreds of intuitive readings in my counseling work, and where there is negative emotion held in the aura, and/or the body, it creates a dark cloud of energy and a corresponding feeling of lack of self-love. This emotion gives rise to all other emotions from fear, grief and even anger. Most people try to find something in the world to fill this loss of love, and they often turn to addictions, not only drugs and alcohol, but money, power, sexuality, etc. But the truth is, only the purposing of the divine within can ultimately fill the loss.

Additionally, when we have negative karma (ignorant actions) from past lives, the Soul brings it forth into the present and creates circumstances and events that allow the individual to recompense errors from the past and provide opportunities to forgive and love ourselves as well.

yourself to the great way, you align yourself to the knowing of where you are going.

The alignment of knowing where you are going is a profound adjustment. It is adjusting the nature of you to a greater way of you. The teacher in you becomes a master student of the Eoma. To be a master student of the Eoma you must be a teacher of many. The many are the ones that give you the credibility to call forth the Eoma.

The next step is to hone imaging. The imagination phase is extremely important. Calling on the Ah-La shows the force of the unseen. The force of the unseen then becomes manipulated by all experience, and when your experience is dictated by your imagination … your great imagining becomes your experience.[102]

The key message of today's reading is that you are the caller. Your students are the re-callers. They call upon you in what you have called upon God. The reason they are going through you on this is so that it can be a planetary experience and not just a spirit experience … for the planet.[103]

All trials on the human plane are a manipulation of the matter … material constructs. Material construct is calling itself forth in vibration. All vibration can be manipulated. The matter, no. The vibration, yes. The vibration gets

---

102   This is a potent statement affirming the power of imagination; when you imagine and feel with clear intention and focus, you create your life circumstances. Feel prosperity, love and joy and it will be so. If dark emotions and feelings surround you, then pain and suffering will be drawn to you.

103   The wave form generated by such a focused and dynamic group transforms the vibration of the planet. It is not about fighting against poverty, disease, social injustice and greed … this increases negative resistance. Transformation occurs when a wave signature of light and love is created. It is like the sun; it doesn't demand that you take your thick overcoat off in its warmth. You give yourself to its embracing warmth and let go. Negativity is dispelled by enlivening the wave form of love that Is at the very basis of all creation, the One light of God.

conditioned from the experience of the Eoma and the experience of the Eoma is then shared from the experience of the teacher, and the students become masters in training.[104]

Gary: When I'm doing the Ujjayi breathing, I can actually feel there is a much larger opening around the heart center, and it begins to feel that the body is calling and breathing the void through the lens of my imagination of the Christ. So, isn't it a breathing from literally inside of everything … spirit exists within all creation, or breathing it out of the void into manifestation?

SOURCE: *That last one, because the void is the attribute of the collection. What you are collecting is the organized form of manifestation. You collect that into you, in your Ujjayi. Then what you express becomes the manipulated form. The form is also the manifest. The manipulated form and manifest then have all opportunity, provided there is some intention. If you begin this in your meditation, you set an intention that might say, in this breathing I will understand there are things coming up that require one hundred percent of me. You then breathe in from the void a calling for the hundred percent of you. When you call for the one hundred percent of you and express this understanding and knowing, then the body starts to feel an understanding of what it's supposed to do, how it is to be, why it is important that it (body) become at one hundred percent of your calling. When you have an intention that is sharing*

---

104 An important teaching here, because trying to change things is hard-won. When we understand that the underlying vibration in all matter contains a perfect blueprint for its ultimate manifestation, then we know the magic of transforming ourselves by creating a new vibrational signature. Moreover, this automatically translates into new awareness and circumstances in the outer reality. The "so called" outer reality is but a mirror of the vibrations within each individual. If there is anger and hatred, even at an unconscious level, then the world appears that way. If there is lack, fear and worry within, then prosperity, joy and peace cannot be found. This is the popularly coined phrase "The Law of Attraction." Rather than trying to attract through manipulation of matter, change your vibration and there is the magic of alchemy.

my experience with my students, you are calling upon the remembrance of all thirty-five years of experience in the great void, when you have been in the void. This void is where you go when you are deep into meditation. You float within the void. And it is in this floating within the void that you identify what is body and what is spirit. Floating in the void, you actually feel the boundaries of your experience, the boundaries of your experience of what you are. When you share this so that others start to feel this, you make your intention; this is the nature of this meditation for me to share my experience with this room. In this room they will feel what I am. In that feeling of what I am, they will expand that part of themselves and understand what I am teaching.

Whenever your intention is for that which is outside of you, you <u>breathe</u> in the void in a greater sense. It must be a greater sense, because it has to expand beyond your body, instead of just curling up within it. It is actually expanding out from the core of you, so it is a vibration that is more like the Doppler radar. It has a rhythm to it, a pattern to it. That pattern is extended from your spine all the way out beyond the room, so that it can enclose the room in your experience. As you feel the calling back through the Ujjayi breathing from your students, you know that's where you are, and you know that is what the intention is for them. Your students can set an intention if you ask them to at that point; they can set an intention that states, in this meditation I am going to discover the part of me I do not understand. When they set the intention and you express your experience, then you are taking them deeper into the ways of themselves.[105]

---

105   The void is the repository of all things possible, waiting to come into manifestation. The inhale of the Ujjayi breath summons all possibilities, but then we must give it an intention in order to create the possibilities we choose. Our intention, along with focus and imagination, causes the Eoma to precipitate substance around our choices, and then spirit gives it life.

Gary: What is the phased shift that takes place in the heart?

SOURCE: *You can think of it as being a pattern similar to a pulsing engine. The heart is the engine of God within the body. When it is pulsing at a normal pace, it is of the human. When it is expressing itself as God, then the phase is a faster pulsing. The heart vibrates at a higher frequency, a faster movement. This faster movement is a holding center. It's not like you are going into a heart palpitation; it is a holding center. Your phase of the knowing of you actually becomes in phase with the knowing of God that is in your heart. When it becomes in-phase, it has shifted phase from human condition to God position.*[106]

Sondra: I love it when God rhymes.

Gary: As I have been doing this very deep Ujjayi breathing over the last month, it feels like my body is being torn up from inside out and restructured, lots of pain everywhere.

SOURCE: *Yes. It won't subside until you have conditioned your body to withstand these new vibrations.*[107]

Gary: An atom is 99.999% space, and so the space would be the void. The electron is surmised as a fuzzy mass of thought, so God was able to circumscribe space, with thought intentionality, and create the holographic universe.

---

106   I was to learn in later sessions that the Christ energy is a whirling, prismatic form of the Star Tetrahedron (Christ Star) which creates an energetic opening in the area of the heart chakra. It is an inter-dimensional doorway back into the realms of Spirit/Void. Truly, the heart is the doorway to God within!

107   This restructuring is an ongoing event as I continue to upgrade the frequency of the body in order to match the Soul's function. A good analogy would be like turning the body into a nuclear reactor. This analogy has some validity because when we see pictures of Jesus, there is often a brilliant light emanating, like the sun, from the heart region.

SOURCE: *Perfect, you have said it exactly so.*[108]

Gary: When one is breathing, one is able to breathe out of every atom in one's body, spirit life.

SOURCE: *Let us correct you there. You breathe into the space between each atomic particle. You become the mover and the manipulator because you breathe into the space between every particle in the universe; this is your intent. It is not possible until you become of the higher stages of spirit. Then you become a creator-being, and all kinds of other things occur in your development. Ultimately, your intent is to express through every phase so that you are aware of every molecule necessary to move you into the direction of your becoming. You are calling on All Being that will take you there.*[109]

Gary: Would that be my will and intention, calling upon that?

SOURCE: *Yes. If you imagine this, it's like looking at someone juggling balloons, and you know how they are floating in the air and hands are moving them upwards, keeping them from falling. That becomes your will. That is your will moving in the spaces between particles.*

---

108   Quantum physics postulates that an electron is a fuzzy mass of energy, sometimes existing as a wave and sometimes as a particle. But metaphysics understands this to be consciousness ... the mind of God circumscribes space.

109   I highlight this paragraph because it would be too easy to overlook this very important and helpful statement: "You are calling on All Being that will take you there." The consciousness of the One pervades the universe. We are the progeny of the One, and like a loving parent, when you beseech your beloved, it hears and responds to your prayer.

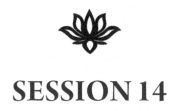

SESSION 14

Effervescence of Spirit

Gary: I had a profound revelation a couple of days ago. When I'm breathing the void, I am actually breathing spirit-life into this dimension. I realized that spirit is actually life force that animates reality. I'm breathing through the life force. As I image it in the Christ lens, it is actually bringing God into form. It's not just spirit, it's not just God, it's actually the life-animating force.

Sondra: It's the animation of life, and without it life can't animate; it's just like dead matter.

Gary: That's right.

Sondra: No matter.

Gary: No matter. Yeah, it's amazing because you realize you become that animating energy which is breath. You are the lens, but you're also seeing what you can be, because you've reflected this through the lens of your consciousness, and so you're the three and the one. You are spirit, mind, body, which is the void, Christ, manifestation.

Sondra: Right, you're the calling of it forth. You're the will of the being.

Gary: You can actually feel it as you are breathing it in. You are the lens and whatever you choose to image and feel is clothed in the possibilities you imagine as the Eoma forms itself around that particular image. If you hold the feeling long enough, then manifestation would literally happen.[110]

SOURCE: *We would call this healing or creating wholeness by knowing the Greater Self that you call through the Eoma. But we would like to share another form of healing that isn't exactly like breathing into the Eoma. It's something different, and it also uses Christ energy; it's something that is a remembrance of a fully healthy body. You breathe in the memory of the healthy body you had before you were in states of pain or discomfort. Before you experienced pain your body was whole. When you breathe into that feeling/image, that's what calls to the Eoma to bring back this nature of full wholeness into the body.*

We use this technique whenever someone is in some kind of difficult torture, not a physical ailment such as a broken leg, because the memory of the leg that was whole doesn't give the healing power to the leg that is broken, because it requires more than what the healed leg knew. The healed leg doesn't know about bringing all of the antibiotics rushing through the leg. The broken leg is a condition where you would want to call forth the Eoma, because it's pulling from all possibilities.[111]

Gary: Understood, but within spirit, isn't the perfect pattern of the Christ already existing?

110　This information had been clearly presented in prior sessions, but when I experienced the feeling in my body it was real beyond disbelief. The mind can know, but until it is felt … it is not so.

111　The precipitation of the Eoma around the Christed image creates materiality. If the body is in stress and pain, and we remember and clearly image the feeling of wholeness, the Eoma reforms the body to that perfect pattern.

SOURCE: *The Christ is not a pattern; it is a style of patterning. It's a way to pattern wholeness. You can have variations on those patterns depending on what you call forth. If you call forth the master of darkness to create the pattern for your power, that's a completely different power structure from what you're working within. When you're working within the power structure that is the Christing nature, this has an effervescence to it that recalls the great redeemer. All great redeemers are in line in the source continuum. They are in line.*

Sondra: What do you mean, in line? How are they in line?

SOURCE: *They are in line to serve, so it's a power structure of line, aligned, service from the straight condition. It's a straight condition ... true straight. The true straight condition requires an essence of knowing what the Christ nature is, and what the patterning condition the Christ nature does. Christ nature patterns itself in the effervescence ... effervescence arising, always arising.[112]*

That's how ascension can occur with a spirit that is following the Christ nature. It is always arising. If you chose to call forth the dark influences, that would be a condition of surface manipulation. You're manipulating the surface of things, so there is an <u>appearance</u> of adjustment. That's how charlatans become powerful, that's how manipulators become powerful magicians. Dark force workers become powerful when they're working in the manipulation of surface. This is a false structure of power. The structure of power of the Christing is working within the deep within to power up into the great ascension, and the alignment of natures that align to that are all Great Masters that have ever worked in this particular power structure. They also align with you as you call it forth. You have multi-dimensional alignment in the Christing nature. Every

---

112   The Christ field is the mystical marriage of divine masculine power and divine feminine love. It is a crystalline structure that is the acknowledgment of Oneness within Source. It patterns only that which upholds and edifies the brilliant way of Source becoming, through its effervescent nature. This is the lineage of all Great Beings who unify and edify the Great Way of God.

time you call it forth, what you're bringing to the effervescence is your memory of you. You retain an attuned nature within the symbols of identity. You will always be Gary Springfield, even after you ascend to higher natures, because that is the name given to you at the point of your acceptance of this. The Gary Springfield is the God are you, bringing forth within a field of all Great Being.[113]

Gary: Is field in this context the Eoma?

SOURCE: *Yes, field is the Eoma.*

Gary: I had an epiphany last night when I woke up at about two a.m. and sat up in bed to meditate. I moved to that place of breathing spirit, life force, in and through. I could feel the body as nothing but spirit. I was the lens of the Christ mechanism, and everything was just a holographic out-picturing of the possibilities of God. It was all a dream that wasn't real. It's not real; in one sense, it's just a holographic imaging. We are consciousness, moving in and through the holographic dream, to sense it and to feel it. But the actual physicality of it is very dreamlike, because it's just ninety-nine-point-nine percent space.

SOURCE: *Correct, this is the effervescence. In the projection that you saw, what you recognized is what God is in spirit, and then matter forms around this imagining power. What you call real, in the three-dimensional field, is actually a system of calling forth what has already been projected. This projection power is what is real. The matter that forms around that projection is being called forth from that real.*

---

113   The Christ field acknowledges the vibration of wholeness that underlies all self-imposed illusions of separateness. This true frequency transmutes from within rather than manipulating the outer form. The master of the Christ condition, Jesus, could see the underlying vibration of Source Oneness within someone, even though they believed in their own disease. His unwavering "Seeing" of God within was a true vibration that re-patterned the surface condition, which was their illusion in separateness. But then he said, "go forth and sin no more," which meant if you revert back to your old ways of ignorance and debauchery, then disease will be yours again.

Gary: Yes, and is that the Eoma?

SOURCE: *Yes.*

Gary: The Eoma would be the glittering substance as well.[114]

SOURCE: *Exactly. It glitters the memory, the memory is the holding ... the memory is a sticky substance, memory, it's a holding, mmmeh, (lips holding together), holding mmmmemory. This is what calls the Soul to solidify what the spirit has imagined.*

Gary: The Soul solidifies what the spirit has imagined.[115]

⚜ ⚜ ⚜

My friend was at this session and had a question.

Friend: I have a question about healing. There is a gentleman who says he heals from a spirit level, which he claims is extremely rare; he says most people are energetic healers, or move energy, or dispel energy on a more physical or Soul level. He says he goes directly to spirit and bypasses the physical and the soul, and that is extremely rare, which is sort of his claim to what sets him apart from other healers. He can delete programs from the past or the future that are not serving you, or keep you stuck.

---

114   All possibilities already exist within the Mind of Source/God. The Christ identifies "the spirit-life" of the "unseen" within the void and images it into manifestation through the effervescent Eoma; Christ is the lens and the Eoma the substance.

115   This struck me as being quite a profound statement. When you say the word "memory" there is the sound of mmmmeh that you pronounce for a moment (lips stuck together) before completing the word, and this is the essence of the Christ holding the image fixed ... mmmmemorizing it (holding together), while the Eoma glitters it into form.

SOURCE: *That part's untrue. The truth that he is working through spirit, yes, absolutely true. But his ability to delete programming can't occur without the individual's acknowledgement of what the programming is. He might remove it in that moment, but then they just reprogram it, because they haven't identified what is programming it.*

Friend: And is it true most healers don't heal from the spirit level and that's a very rare gift?

SOURCE: *Yes, it is, but that doesn't mean he's more effective than those that work within the Soul level. The Soul is always trying to move spirit deeper into the body. It's a constant communication. When you work with the Soul, and you relieve tension between the Soul and the body, because the body recognizes the Soul ... the Soul calls forth and serves spirit. This is what he is doing. Within you is this same ability to move spirit into the body in any given manner of healing. It's always a conditioning where someone is removing a block, even if just temporarily to bring your attention to what you've felt healed.*

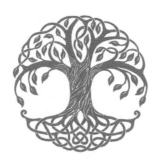

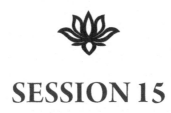

SESSION 15

The Mountain Is Not The Goal

Gary: Is there anything that I can do right now to further serve the work?

SOURCE: We want you to focus on the trials of your worthy way and separating from the trials of your students. You have a course that is going to need you to shed some of the burden of your students in a way that doesn't make them feel abandoned, but will make them see you in a different light. The way you can start seeing them is by transitioning your process from strain to gain. The strain is the one that tries to bridge, that tries to help, and the one that tries to hold. This is the you that is wanting company in your place of the path. But the company that you're going to keep is a shamanic form of Sherpas, the ones that go with the mountain climbers, the ones that aid them in the climb. These are the kinds of students you're going to start acquiring, and these Sherpas will be able to make the climb with you because they've already strayed from the pack a long time ago. They've strayed from that which would have held them in the world, although they didn't do it in a way that kept them from interacting with the world. They did it in a way that kept the world at bay while they continued what they needed to do in order to survive in the world. These people have done everything necessary to maintain their abundance at a level that sheds emotional trials along the path. Many of your students are still dealing with emotions, and until they shed that, they just can't go beyond the mountain.[116]

The mountain is not the goal, the mountain is the source of your climb. It is what gives you altitude … although it is not that which you are seeking. Many people see the mountain as the thing to conquer, but the conquering is their own fear, their own shame and unworthiness. When they are able to see their transition in that way, then that's what they focus on, and they are perfectly fine with a simple life. Many of your students are not fine with the simple life, yet they have no idea how to have anything but a simple life. They are illogical in their way of addressing it, and illogical in their way of showing their worth. They continue to look for things in the world to give them a source of happiness, or a source of fulfillment. They want a good job that pays them a lot of money and make them happy. They want a system that makes it possible for them not to work and focus only on their spiritual life. They may want a relationship so they can feel good about themselves so they can have the kind of life they think they're supposed to have when working for God. So many things that people want in their life have nothing to do with the spirit they're seeking.[117]

꧁ ꧁ ꧁

---

116   I was introduced to the new information about the Christing way only 10 months ago, and I can see at this juncture how I had been wanting to pull students and friends along on the path, because I cherish each and every one of them. However, spirit is letting me know this is impossible when someone has not done the work and/or is unwilling to do the work.

117   There is nothing wrong with an individual seeking fulfillment in the world, while at the same time enjoying their modest excursions into their spiritual life. Some folks are not ready, willing or able to go through the deep work to clear the emotional body and learn to love themselves. No judgment, but the path of the Great Way of forging union with the divine is arduous, demanding and committed.

We never expected the One Hundred to come to fruition until such time that individuals have made certain strides. We see where those strides need to be in order for them to maneuver in the circles you are going to be in. We know this is a minimum of a three-year journey just to have a foundation of the One Hundred. We aren't in any way concerned with the speed. The only thing we are concerned with now is that you have the ability to shed this desire to bring everyone with you. We want more than anything for them to all come, but they can't, because they won't, and they won't because they aren't. That's the only thing stopping them … what they will and won't do. What they will, is that which the world tells them is acceptable. Even though it seems as if they're doing just the opposite, the only reason they're doing the opposite in their doing is because what they see is something frightening, but they still want it. So they try to journey within it from a spiritual bubble, but that bubble needs to go within their heart and within their own being, not outside of them protecting them from the world. It needs to be within them so that protection is with them everywhere, including the very difficult steps of journeying into the world.[118]

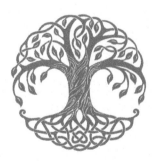

---

118   The gist of this session was to help me understand that the foundation of the One Hundred, spoken about it Session 5, is happening but there needs to be a culling, refinement and refocus on my part. This will allow the people who choose themselves, the necessary time to come together, and the skillfulness to climb together. This will assure the foundation of the One Hundred develops organically, like a multi-petaled flower.

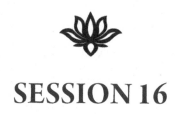

SESSION 16

Imagination Creates

Gary: Is there any information today about the next step on my path?

SOURCE: *Don't be distracted by the world. Hold within you that which is your responsibility, and it is always about understanding the Christing way. The Christing way is an everlasting expression of you. The leadership of the Christing way requires that you stay on track with the nature of the Christ. If you get off track with other messages, then people get confused about what you're all about. We have to keep you in line with the Christing way, or we cannot identify for you what are your next steps.*[119]

The structure of this requires that you pull in the power of the universe and then express it through yourself. That's why you are so adamant about what people see deep within their meditation and their body, because you know the

---

[119]   When I first started meditating in 1976, I was fascinated about the "Christ" from my extensive metaphysical readings and studies in college. Like so many others, I thought that "Jesus Christ" was the transfigured man. I knew his words, "What I have done all men can do" were possible and true. I did not understand until now that it's a system of patterning wholeness within … with Source Oneness. These sessions were about preparing me to understand and embody this truth so I could share these revelations. My dedication to the path of enlightenment has always been supreme, and so I became ever more dedicated, disciplined and focused in order to create the optimum experience for myself and for others.

sense of the cell is what is the condition of the Christ. You don't have words for it; you don't know how to use it, but this is what you know in a knowing. You're going to learn how to make it a being. In this making of a being, you're going to have words as you feel into the feeling of the being.

The cellular process that goes on is just like respiration. If you look up the word respiration, you will learn what it says about what's happening in the cells through respiration. You'll start to identify what is the calling forth of the Christing of the cells of the body.

There's no way to change cells, what you're doing is changing the environment of the cells. You change what is outside of the cells by giving a whole new planetary adjustment. This planetary adjustment relates to the perspective of the individual; you alter their perspective. If you alter their perspective by the nature of your being, you create a new environment and cells create themselves based on that environment.

Cells create themselves in the environment of something new and worthy. When they are in states of unworthiness, they repel that which is their best thing; these cells cannot believe it's true. When you place them in an environment where they forget what they believe, then they alter based on the environment and adapt to survive. They adapt to survive in order to "be" that which is the environment they're in, because that is the nature of evolution. Evolution evolved to understand the environment.

When you change the environment, you are a creator-being. As a creator-being, you create the environment for each cell to make what they are and what they want to be. Cells can only be what they want to be when you take them out of the environment that's making them what they are.[120]

The only way to replenish is to pull in the Christing nature that is redemption. It's calling in the floods of emotion that will destroy all that is no longer, which means the remnants of the past finally get destroyed by the replenishing of the redemption of the wholeness of the Christing way within the body. Pulling it in, journeying within, holding it there and elevating it to the high, high, high. The elevation of is a calling forth, Ahhhhhhhhh-Laaaaaaaaa, and all that are called are relieved when they <u>know</u> what they are calling for. When they don't know what they're calling for, then they just keep calling, and that's the cancer. Cancerous cells keep calling and calling. But Intention, intention is what you're training people in their call. They call themselves forth and understand what they are, so give them something to intend. You can give them all kinds of options; your intention today, maybe, you meet your greater being within and ask it, where are you now and where are you going?

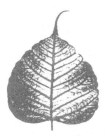

120   The statement that evolution is about adapting to the environment is how all evolution on Earth has transpired. It is not a process of life-forms developing from within, it is life adjusting to a new environment for survival. Equally important, the mind and the feeling nature of an individual can create a new environment with imagination. You focus inner light upon the image/feeling which creates a new feeling environment. Dr. Bruce Lipton does fascinating work with epigenetics, which is the sequencing of new DNA structures within the body by altering environments. It was once thought that the inherited patterns in our DNA could not be altered except through random disorder, but epigenetics has proven otherwise.

These options are endless in the supply of intention, so long as each individual gives themselves an intention … pursuing the love of their own being. Pursuing it in joy, wondering who am I, what am I, where am I, what can I be?[121]

Gary, this is why the evolution of your being has to keep moving forward; if you fall backward and rely on that which you read instead of that which you experience, then you no longer have the experience to teach. Some individuals only teach that which someone else experienced, and that is not teaching. That is simply disseminating someone else's information. There are people whose job it is to do that, but not you. Your job is to experience and reveal, experience and reveal, and every time you reveal, your students experience that new fullness.

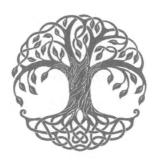

---

121   The Christ within calls into the Eoma to manifest the wholeness, which the Christ holds in imagination. When the ego is calling from a place of lack and self-derision, consciously or even unconsciously, the calling is a confusing, incoherent vibration that causes the cells and tissues in the area of the body holding derision to become cancerous. This is the body's attempt to get attention; disease is the "calling" from within, beseeching the individual to look at the derision, and call wholeness and love into being. The Christ system changes the environment by feeling love and peace within and creates a true healing. Allopathic medicine tries to alter the cells, which is difficult and often futile in many diseases. Medicine and surgery can provide a temporary fix, but if the individual has not altered their belief, the cancer comes back; disease surfaces again because the internal environment did not change. When your intention is the love of your own being, pursuing your joy, wondering what can I be, you are patterning the Great Way of wholeness within.

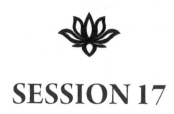

SESSION 17

Environmental Shift

Gary: What is the next teaching that I should bring forth?

SOURCE: *We are building an understanding in you of the Christed way, which is ancient. In its ancient nature there is very little in the modern world that will understand it. Everything you get from us with regard to the Christed way has to be adopted, adapted, and memorized. It has to be brought into your way of being, because we are bringing you step-by-step into an understanding that is absolutely critical for your life's work.*

You were put on this planet for one important reason, and that is to bring the Christed way to the people in a manner that becomes more intrinsic to the way people think about the body, mind, spirit combination, rather than the current Jesus Christ myth.

The Jesus Christ myth is too pervasive, and it has brought many people to their knees due to lack of understanding. There needs to be someone leading the way, and Gary you were designed to lead this way. It is a condition you were designed to understand and teach. In your mastery you must teach it, for if not, you will not have served your greatest way. It's only in the brand-new awareness of ideas that the body actually begins to break itself down in a gentle way the old ideas and misinformation.

A master must focus one's life only on their mastery if one is to become the master (master simply means teacher). You were designed to be the teacher of the Christed way, the mastery of the Christed way. It is a condition that human beings do not understand, and the more they think they understand Jesus Christ, they lose the point of the nature of the Christ.

When students lose the point of the nature of the Christ, they start to identify with idolatry. This is something that occurs in every generation; i.e., some form of idolatry. Whether it is idolizing the nature of some condition of utopia, idolizing a condition of the nature of God embodied in some person, or if it's in some way of being that people generate their own adoption of, and think that this is the correct and only way to go.

There is a fine line between idolatry and understanding the nature of a given message. The message is adopted; it is not registered. The false idea is, "This is the registration of the way of God and God only, and any other forms of registration will not work." Your mastery and the messages being given to you are not registered for anyone else but you. You are a master of this, and others choose to follow in your path because they want to understand the greater way of it.

As you fall deeper into the greater way of it, you bring people with you, and they observe it within their own way of observation. But you become it, and they observe you becoming it, and wonder, "What is it in me that is my great mastery that I am to become?" You go deeper into your becoming of the Christed way. You go deeper into your becoming of the nature of the Christ. You become this wellspring you were born to be.[122]

Now you have to go into the knowing. It's time for you to understand knowing. Knowing is a course, and it is a course that you must understand in the Christed way. All knowing is unique with each individual. Each individual has knowings and words that are abundant within them as they describe more and more the mountain that they are. And you are describing more and more the mountain that you are in the Christed way.

If students idolize you for your wisdom, you create a form of Soul entrapment, because they have no way to be other than how you say they are to be. You must show them the source of your own being, and that source is in God being.

Your course is an understanding of what knowing is beyond thinking. Knowing that thinking is not the same as knowing. Knowing is full being, but it is full being in word and deed. Knowing is a deed. It is how you do what you do because you have justification for it in your knowing. What you know is profoundly important and has come much from your being.

---

122   The original and authentic teaching, given to the disciples of Jesus in the Essene schools, was the understanding that the Christ is the patterning of creation. The Christ system opens the doorway into the void. The "Father" (spirit) is summoned in order to infuse spirit/life into the knowing, which the Christ holds in the acknowledgment of Source/God. The religious idolatry in the time after Jesus bastardized this truth for the sake of priestly power, and claimed it was only through the church that God could be found ... but never embodied ... because Jesus was the savior who died for their sins.

This new understanding cannot be idolized and registered as the only way. The way is within all humans when they create self-love and coherence within, and step upon the self-empowered path of the Great Way. This will be understood as the Christ field, the creative mechanism of the universe, not a singular person.

It is more than belief; knowing is what dictates your will. Your will moves forward in an unconscious manner. Will is not a conscious thing, it is a force of will, this is not will. Will is its own wave, and it moves through you based solely on your knowing. Your knowing is a programmed way, unless you alter the default. When you alter the default, it means you are highly conscious. And you're teaching consciousness in others so they can alter their own default and understand the mechanism for making things.

The mechanism for making things is high in the holding of the way of Christ. In this highest way is the Eoma. But in the Eoma there is total chaos; it's just "all things possible." The Christed way is the acknowledgment of all things possible, in order to disintegrate that which traps you. The Christed way says to your knowing: I know all things are possible, and in that knowing all things are possible, I remove myself from this understanding that is trapping me. When I remove myself from what is trapping me and acknowledge all things are possible, it's through the Christed way I start to call that which I desire. That which I desire starts to formulate in me an understanding of what the new direction is so that I become the full bounty of that which I was born to be. When I become the full bounty of that which I was born to be, I follow the path of the Christed way telling me over and over again all things are possible right now.[123]

---

123   This is an important acknowledgment that for most individuals their will power is an unconscious program that has been imposed upon them through parental, cultural, and societal programing. There is no judgment in this fact, because it was the choice each Soul made when they incarnated. When you become conscious of the Great Way, and acknowledge the Christ condition within, you change the old default program into a conscious knowing, "This is my intention and way." This new way dissolves old programs that keep you trapped and bound in limitation.

All things are possible. "So, what's possible in this moment?" you ask the Christed way. And the Christed way tells you what's possible, what's in the light, what is the light here, what light am I missing in this moment of misery, where is the light in this, show me. The Christed way shows you and you acknowledge this is the way out. This is the way out of the entrapment. This is the way of my knowing, full well my knowing. Condition me only in the Christed way, and in the Christed way my condition becomes an alleviated way.

The alleviated way acknowledges that all things are possible because the Eoma is all I need to acknowledge in order to make all that is possible come alive. It comes alive in me. I am profoundly abundant in what it's trying desperately to recreate in me when I forget who I am. When I forget, I know the first thing I need to be is a profound abundance of me. This is the totality of the world around me, because it is all that I see.[124]

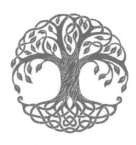

124 The Eoma is all things possible within the chaos. The Christ system identifies the all things possible in the knowing, and with the intention for wholeness it summons spirit/void to fill-full this pattern/image. When you choose to only see abundance and peace, your knowing of the Christ brings prosperity and peace into your reality. Within the Christ field, physical healing, the manifestation of loaves and fishes and all things possible are true. "Ask, and it will be given to you; seek, and you will find; knock, and the door will be opened to you." Matthew 7:7.

SESSION 18

Star Particle

SOURCE: *We want to give you some extra terrain to develop in your mind on how to encompass the nature of the Christed way and provide some parameters to people with regard to how to understand it.*

The first parameter is that people need to know the Christed way is an ancient and abundant stellar strength, as in the stars. It is a strength of manifestation that produces the stars.

The Christed way is in stardust; every speckle of dust contains an effervescent condition that began from a solar polisus. Polisus is impossible for us to describe at this point, but just know that it is a process, and it is a condition of a star.

The condition of a star is holding the Christed way, because the star develops from the Eoma. A star is created in the purposeful consciousness that is the Christed way. The condition of the Christ for the purpose of our working

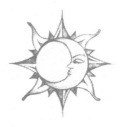

through you, Gary, on Earth ....[125]

Sondra: Excuse me, I missed what was said. Did you just say the condition of the Christ on Earth?

SOURCE: *Yes, the condition of Christ on Earth. The reason why we are working through Gary to develop a Christed way, it is his daemonship. A daemonship isn't a demon as in devil demon. It is a Daemon, which is a Greek word meaning genius. So, it is a genius within the individual that comes alive when one begins to understand their true calling. Once that true calling kicks in, then the daemon is the parameter of the individual who conditions themselves in their own way of being, or the way they were created from. In that creating comes an understanding of one's daemon. Gary's particular daemon is with regard to the Christed way. In this parameter, what Gary's going to show, is the stellar, ancient stellar way of being created. It's a stellar way of creating.*

---

125   In the original star formation of the universe eons ago, hydrogen gas spiraled and coalesced into form, then ignited into a nuclear radiance. These first stars burned themselves out after billions of years and collapsed upon themselves with such a force of gravity that the hydrogen and helium molecules were pressed together with such tremendous pressure that this created all the dense molecules such as oxygen, iron, carbon, etc. When the stars exploded it spewed these elements out into space. When a new star birthing began, which is similar to our galaxy, the birthing star was able to gather this mineral dust and create planets. The physical, you and I, are made of this mineral substance which also formed the Earth, and so every particle within you is stardust! The Soul we are animates this "stardust." We are stardust in motion, living on a planet in order to realize the God being we are that created the whole shebang to see itself. It's all US!

Sondra: The Christed way?

SOURCE: *Yes. The stellar way of creating. You're going to explain to students that stars are made from the Christed way. Stars are an abundance of the nature of Christ calling forth from the Eoma in an organized fashion so that the star itself can create planets and planets create life. This condition of the Eoma into an organized ball of fire is what we want people to recognize as the source of their energetic core.*

The source of their energetic core comes from the same place that a great star born out of the Eoma comes from. The only way they're able to identify with themselves in a way that says, I am God, I make things, I can make my world whatever I want it to be, is when they call upon the Christing order within themselves that organizes the chaos of the all things possible into something they can materialize in their life. How they call on that is in various ways, but in particular, we've called upon it in our session together with the breathing, the Ah-La, and the call of the void that Gary does.[126]

The second parameter is about the facility of the Christed way. The only way to be a facility of the Christed way is to understand that the Eoma is all things possible. It may seem chaotic because it contains all that is, and all that ever was, but within that containment is a select story. A select story comes from an emotional way. The emotional way that creates the story of the life of an individual is the story they tell themselves and they tell others. They tell this story over and over again until such time that it becomes them, and the story is them, and that story retells them within whatever environment they're in. They retell the story of the story that's telling them.

But when you create the strength of an individual by changing the default of

---

126   The Christ field identifies what's next within the all things possible and coalesces this pattern into manifestation through the Eoma. Individuals can begin to master the Christ system when they learn how to breathe in spirit, from the infinite void, through the open doorway within.

the old story, you give them new parameters to become the story of abundance and joy. The alternate is to tell the story that you become, that tells the story of your becoming. The way that is to be seen in relation to the Eoma, is that the Eoma is a story-driven keeitofreeshen.[127]

Sondra: Okay, what's a keeitofreeshen?

SOURCE: *It's impossible to translate that word, impossible. But here's the gist of it. Keeitofreeshen is the connection between the Eoma and the Christed way. You can imagine the Christed way as a river in the mountain, and that river draws whatever is next to it into the water, and it goes down the stream. It is the downstream condition of a river that is aligned with the understanding of the Eoma related to the Christed way. Christed way being the river that runs that which is in the Eoma down to that which is the calling of it. It is a river running to that which calls. How that calls is what each individual has to understand with regard to their story. The story is the calling; calling what is necessary to make that story real. Each story that's told has a real nature because the Eoma has responded through the Christing way.*

Sondra: Even if it's a tumultuous story or a story of why the victim?

SOURCE: *No, no, no, just the opposite. The story that one tells that is a way of being the ceremonial self-awareness is the one that we are talking about here, which is related to the Christed way. Otherwise, the story that an individual tells*

---

127   So few people understand that what they believe and feel about themselves is their story, and if their story is based upon beliefs of limitation, fear, worry and self-derision this unconsciously summons from the Eoma the all things possible as pain, suffering and lack. This morose condition then retells their story by their continual acknowledgment of the pain, suffering and derision they experience, and is compounded by the things they judge and criticize in the world. When you step upon the path of the Great Way, you know you can tell the story of abundance and wholeness through the Christed system, (and through the Keeitofreeshen, so eloquently explained in the next paragraph) the new reality is created.

that makes them a victim becomes that which is the body's own interpretation of a story … its own interpretation of the world around it, and of itself. It's a destructive story. An instructive story takes the Christed openness, calls forth from the Eoma what is necessary to become and moves down river into the way of the self-aware.

The self-aware tells a new story. The new story is, "I am abundant and every abundance that I am is calling forth through the I Am. And through the I Am is an awareness that there is nothing that I cannot be, nothing that I will not do, and nothing that I cannot work through." It doesn't mean that each person who calls forth this manifest destiny is without strife, it just means that that strife is not an inward derision, it's an external strengthening. It brings character to a life, rather than destruction.[128]

The third parameter for the conditions of the Christed way is the stolen nature. The stolen nature is when an individual feels as if they have been robbed of an essential condition; i.e., they've been robbed of good parents, parents at all, did not receive unconditional love, the world owes them, or the universe owes them in some way. Anyone who is in a condition of entitlement is also someone who is experiencing the stolen way. These are spoiled brats with regard to spiritual development. They are brats and they need to be addressed when it comes to teaching the Christed way. The Christed way requires a maturity of one's spirituality. The maturity is all about what has been surrendered to make. What has been given to develop you, and who has made sacrifices to

---

128   In this analogy of the keeitofreeshen, the Christ identifies, within the "ocean" of all possibilities, a particular feeling/image of wholeness. The focused attention the Christ holds with that thought/image is symbolic of the "living-waters" of the river that flow unwavering towards that possibility. The Christ holds the "focused-way" which summons and gathers the substance from the riverbank, the soil and minerals of the Eoma, to manifest and make real the image. As we adopt the Christed way, we learn to flow as the "living river." We can experience difficulties along the way, but these build strength and character, rather than disturbance.

create the story that you need to reinterpret. The brats that get into a spiritual movement, because it is the only way they feel comfortable in the world, because they cannot maneuver in the world without this constant reassurance that everything is fine, and they're fine, and the world is fine, and there is nothing wrong with anything, it's just your interpretation of things, and so they suckle on that condition. The way these individuals destroy the nature of the Christ is by interpreting what is supposed to be their service to others into how this can serve them. Even the great masters suffer from moments of disillusionment when it comes to helping others. There's always a drawback to doing that, there is a loss of personal space, there's a loss of time, of personal health and rest, when service to others becomes greater than the service to self. A master sees this as an opportunity to grow, an opportunity to build boundaries, and an opportunity to develop an inner constitution that determines what the road is really going to be like. A brat, however, looks at these as reasons why they are not on the right course. "Well, I can't do this because this has happened to me," rather than, "I'm working through this ... this is the next thing in my learning path; I'm understanding this thing about me."

Now there are some brats in Gary's group. These brats are not to be singled out. They are to be bettered. There are conditions where it works its way out, but in a parameter for teaching the Christed way. What we want you to acknowledge, Gary, is there are going to be people who just cannot move on with you. We know we've told you this before, but the trail of their remiss continues, and this is not your fault. This isn't anything you've done or what anyone else has done. It's just that once the Christing manner of teaching goes full swing, if these people are still in the group, they will sicken themselves. You cannot call upon these great spiritual powers and bring them into you while you are in self-pitying straits. Self-pitying straits, while in the presence of great spiritual abundance, causes an inner severance, because the spirit of you knows what's right. The spirit of you is severed from the being of you when you're in a state of being a brat in the master's course.[129]

Sondra: So, Gary, when I was talking to God about you, what I saw was that you were going to eventually create an energy-vortex gathering in the Christed way?

SOURCE: *Yes, eventually you will start to build the practice of positioning people in a room so that energy flows around, up, and through, and that means nothing with regard to what you're doing now, but eventually this is what you're going to be creating, an energy flow around, up, and through. This energy flow around, up, and through requires that you have people who are of the higher conditioned strengths, pulled back from those who are in the lower vibrational worries. They're in the lower vibrational worries because they don't know how to let go enough for flow to occur around them.*

Sondra: I'm seeing it as a riverbank, and the people who are in the higher spiritual order are on the riverbank, and the ones who are less aware are further inland?

SOURCE: *That's a good way of looking at it. Further inland is away from the flow, away from the riverbank, away from the Christed way. Christed way must be a pure way, and in the pure way that you will energetically create, there is a clear communication soulful nature. The soulful nature is each individual in the room will feel clear communication throughout their whole body. And what they are drawing toward them will be heightened in its expressions with the amount of flow that's flowing around them; it's a manifest heaven. This is what heaven is, this flowing way of all that you think you are, and all that you strive to become. This is heaven. When you open up the Christed way, you are literally*

---

129   As it says here, high vibrational energy begins to cause issues within an individual's spirit and their health if they cannot match the high frequency energy of a dedicated group. I also find these people are not usually called to such an event, and so we can surmise that spirit is directing opportunities from a place of Higher awareness.

holding court for heaven to flow through, around, among, up and to.[130]

This is the last of the needing to know for now. In the course of this needing to know, remember the three parameters. The three parameters are:

—First, the stellar nature, the stellar nature of the Eoma
and the Christed way working together.

—The second is the story, storytelling.

—The third is the perfect alignment confluence.

Gary: When working with the Eoma, as one could fully imagine or image/feel and hold that image and feeling, and breath through it, the Eoma would have to gather itself around that purposeful image/feeling that is held with intentionality to become manifest?

SOURCE: *The intentionality and holding that you are describing is the Christing. The Eoma is simply responding to the Christing. The Eoma is stupid, really; it can't do, say, be anything. It just holds everything that is possible within it. So it has no real consciousness about itself, but it is conscious of that which calls to it. So it becomes an awareness of itself, the minute it hears its own call.*

Gary: So I should also be teaching the feeling and imaging to create one's reality?

SOURCE: *We don't suggest imaging because imaging starts to cause the imagination to have some expectation about what things will look like. What we would suggest, then, instead of creating imaging, is that you create a*

---

130   The energy vortex created would look like a peaceful whirlwind. In the center would be the pure silence of the Christ field summoning the Oneness of spirit from out of the void; manifesting spirit-light though the Eoma. As it flowed around, up and through, it would become more enlivened with the light of those gathered. It is this high vibrational signature that resonates within the higher dimensions and sanctions the essence of the "Heaven on Earth" experience.

feeling of what it looks like, not a vision of what it looks like. The feeling of what something looks like will contain wide-open soul-full natures. The Soul doesn't have the ability to see anything. The Soul can just experience the joy of everything. The Soul's <u>inability</u> to see the imagination of the human brain is a perfect alignment to the way to create something that has the right feeling about it. For instance, you can fall in love with someone and be the perfect match with someone who's never been someone you would imagine. You would have never imagined Jennifer to be the one and only. The mistake of imagining can be altering what the true course is.

Gary: OK, I understand that. I encourage people not to fixate on the image, but more the feeling essence and let Spirit create the image to then manifest it.

SOURCE: *Perfect. Let Spirit create the image. Those are perfect words, we love those words, letting Spirit create the image.*

Gary: In my own Christing feeling in meditation, I feel myself emanating sunlight from inside out, and feel myself golden and radiant. I hold that feeling/image and allow the Eoma to gather itself into what is creating my informed body. Is that right?

Sondra: I'm personally transformed by you describing that.

SOURCE: *Well, the beauty of it, Sondra, is the condition that he is describing. In the condition that Gary describes, you're thinking, wow, I want some of that. And that's the perfection that his genius is. This is his daemon, the creation of the golden beam, the beam of light that beams through you and to you and for you and of you. This is the golden way, and in this golden way is a story, the Christed way. This is your story. This is your making, your perfect becoming. There are people who will be able to observe it in you, and then by conditioning, start to recognize it in glimpses.*

You can teach what the light is we give. We give this light through you and then people experience it from you. In the room, what's created is the vortex of that condition. Because you are emanating this great illumination, and in this emanation of illumination, the sparkle within each individual is responding. And in that response comes the flow of it. It's like temperatures on the surface of the oceans; there are warm spots and cold spots. The warm spots meet cold spots and wind happens. You are this warm glow thumbing upon a wave of coolness, and the flow that is created is the whole shebang (all of it).

These people who are the cold ones have to be clear and pure, in a sense. They can't be cold because they're closed. They're cold because they have their fervent nature focused in other areas of their spiritual life. You become a complement to everything they're already doing in their life, and it rushes across them. Rushes across, like the wind across blades of grass.[131]

Gary: What is the tension I am feeling around my Christing work?

SOURCE: *You're always wanting to solve people's conditions and we love you for that, but it's time for you to try to release where you keep straining yourself. Over time, as you reduce your sense of responsibility for other people's striving or not striving, you let go of them. It's something your inner being wants everyone to be, everyone to be the highest of their spiritual way. Of course, that's what you want, every master does. As the master you are now, you cannot align yourself with what others do or don't do, even if it's true that they should be where you recommended. And so your physical stress is responding to your attempts to be the light for all.*

Gary: I have to be like the sun; the sun shines but doesn't really care if people grow or not, it just shines.

SOURCE: *That's right. Know that those who recognize it will shine.*

---

131   It is a fact in meteorology that when warm air meets cold air, it creates an energetic movement of wind. The spirit breeze we create together will be filled with light, love and transformation.

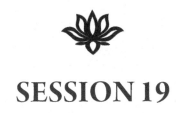

SESSION 19

Christ-Mass

Sondra: I'm curious about the Christmas message.

Gary, you are feeling an upgrade that is starting to have either moments of weighted-ness to it, and then you have to go in to lighten it, because it is too weighty for its system of lightness that takes you into a euphoric mode. The euphoria mode, you will start to see, has a holographic condition to it; you start to see what's being built in your own imaging. This is the articulation of you, understanding the Christening of you. You see how the euphoria is turning life into a holographic view where you are walking through the hologram and seeing every human being that's going to be in this wave with you; knowing exactly why each individual you take into the One Hundred is going to be there. They are articulating a snowflake, this gigantic, beautiful snowflake that reflects the essence of God. The essence in a way that vibrates it into a brilliant shape, a shape we've shown you so far to be like the Merkabah. We've shown you to be like the Ahhh ... Laaa. The Ahhh ... Laaa creates the cell resonance in the shape of the flower of life; cells resonating into a state of their own vibratory manner for a perfection in their replication. More and more you're going to see how these shapes have been in your life before, you just didn't know where they belonged.

The knowing where they belong is going to help you devise your pulling into your life a wholeness, a creator-ness, an Ah-La-ness.[132]

Gary: During meditation, in the third eye there is a clear diamond emanating golden liquid Christing energy, creating an environment for the body to become literally the body of the Christ consciousness.

SOURCE: *The diamond in the auric field is individuating the light, and the many facets of the diamond create the light that is able to transcend what is the individual. An individuated nature of the Christ creates a calling. The calling that is pulled through the individual's field of facets is their fallentation. The fallentation is someone's conditioning for creating the facets of their particular diamond. This is just a metaphor to describe how each individual has created and cut their own siring. To sire oneself is how one births one's own ability to call upon the Christing manner. In the siring of the self, there is a crystallizing of the tension. That crystallizing of the tension is a creation of a diamond, but it really is the holographic nature of finally understanding life to be that which you created it to be.*

---

132   I really loved this feeling of an energetic snowflake imaging the essence of God. The science of cymatics is the study of the creation of matter through sound; the One Hundred would be a cymatic-style vibration of Christedness.

Source also mentioned, for the first time, the Merkabah. Over the next several years, I came to the great realization that this was the star tetrahedron that, when formulated, opens the inner doorway into the void and holds the energy of the Christing experience. As the star tetrahedron spins in all directions it appears as a sparkling golden diamond, which is the Ah-La, the creative sound of God.

And in that is a cutting of your own diamond; it's a literal cutting into and making of what would be your perfect light-gathering method for internalizing the Christing.[133]

When people begin to see that, then the whole world they lived in never again appears. Because suddenly they see a window into what is the nature of God seeing God.[134]

Gary: In one of the readings, Source talked about the sun, the solar logos energy. Are there any further parameters around that statement?

SOURCE: *Yes. Solar Logos is the nature of understanding that the sun is the source of all life. All systems of the sun represent the systems of God. All systems of the sun also represent the way of mankind and his intelligence, and it represents the way the body is in the form of its own intelligence from the sun.*

The sun has so much life in it that it actually gives life to that which has no life, if it recognizes the life. The lifeless human being that walks around with their under manner showing is only in need of their own light. The Solar Logos is the nature of that light and is a way of looking at the principal nature of all that lives. All that lives understands that light is the only source of life, and the only source of life that is light, systematizes that which is the life of

---

133   Initially, I did not make the connection regarding the facets of the diamond and the facets of the star tetrahedron as being the energy signature of the Christ wave. In my meditation and spiritual revelations years later, I realized this Star jewel (Star tetrahedron) was a wave-form created through focused consciousness and light. As it whirled within the auric field it opened a sacred doorway within the heart chakra, back into the realms of the void; i.e., Source/God. From within the "open way" there was a living spring arising forth as the breath of spirit. When I had this revelation, I began to truly understand how these source talks were creating a picture puzzle, piece by piece, of illumination.

134   When the interior doorway opens back into the realms of Source/God, it is God seeing you and you seeing God as One-Being looking at One's Self; I Am That I Am. In the ancient Sanskrit language of India this translates to So'Ham.

the light. If someone understands the Solar Logos of themself, they also get an identity for the way they can live life on the sunny side of the street. This is what your work will eventually remind people, Gary, because you are solar way, a lighted way.[135]

Gary: Is there anything at this time that I can do to further deepen into the Christ consciousness?

SOURCE: *The Christ consciousness is deepening you at this point. The wave of it is working through the articulation of you. You articulate more and more within the understanding of yourself how these things said about you are true. The primary concern for you has always been, how is it that I could be such a thing of great beauty? How could I be something so profound and important? When all my life I've fought to undue the unworthiness I've felt. You're telling me that all this time, not only was I not unworthy, but I was worthy of more than I could even imagine. The articulation of you is what's going on right now. The more you embody it, the more it becomes you and you become it, the more you start to feel a responsibility for it. That's when the real identity is going to have some alteration, and that's when you'll call upon the Christing every single day.*

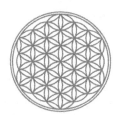

---

135   Our sun and all stellar orbs in the galaxy are emanations of a magnificent Christed being. The word Logos translates as, "The word of God or divine order." And, of course, the light of the sun purposes all life on Earth … it is the light of life.

Even though you are doing it in a way that's more systematic right now, you're identifying that this is the way that it's supposed to be, the need for you to move forward, and you do it incrementally, and it absorbs you as you do it incrementally. [136]

Gary: Are there subtle, vital airs that can be breathed into the head to enliven the self?

Gary Comments: This question elicited a "story" from Source about survival in the future by learning how to "compost" the old and transform it into vital nutrients. Sonda and I both laughed heartily when we understood this was the "job" of the worm.

SOURCE: *The condition of this is wild. It is the wild. So, find in your mind the way of understanding the habitat untouched by mankind. The wild of nature— that's what we mean by wild. It has evolved into its own form of survival. It uses that which is around it as a resource for its survival. In that survival it becomes more abundant. It doesn't question whether or not it's going to survive the wild nor ask if it's going to survive, it just survives.*

When international systems start to become so overt that they destroy all that is wild, there is a loss of the wild. In that loss of the wild, there has to be those airs that are articulated in the breathing. They must be conscious, because the underlying consciousness of it is God, but mankind has forgotten God. The world has absolutely consumed it, so there's nothing left of the wild. There are

---

136   I had been meditating for 35 years with great discipline and dedication when I began this new process being systematically laid out in these dialogues. The information felt profound and true, and equally important, it acknowledged my unwavering love for what I thought was the Christ at that time. I was 100% willing and delighted to give myself over totally to this process, but it sounded daunting and far-reaching. (As I am editing this session it has been 7 years into the work, and I can feel my body, my consciousness and my knowing deepening every day, and I give myself over more and more to the possibility.)

patches left, but there is nothing truly wild to the senses anymore. People don't live in the wild. There's no way to smell it, taste it, touch it; it's all manipulated. It's all brought to a composted system.[137]

The wild, in the way of the calling of the airs, sanctions the body to be pure in the whole. In the wholeness of this, one has to be the worm to be the highest order.

Sondra: We have to be without a nose, eyes, and ears?

SOURCE: *Correct. Everything that is working you, is what you are working through. And as you work through it, you see that your job is partially to a pusher.*

Sondra: A pusher, pusher, you push the dirt around. You're pushing the compost around. I was picturing a worm pushing the dirt around, a pusher.

SOURCE: *No, but we like the image that you created.*

(Much laughter by both Gary and Sondra about the pushing worm.)

SOURCE: *A pusher in the way that we are saying it is an "up" ... u ... p ... upusher; it is a way of ushering in, not pushing out. Ushering in, so you usher in as a worm when you allow the nutrients of that compost to come through it in order to nourish you. The nourishment of the wild that is brought through*

---

137   Source, once again, mentions the difficulties ahead for humanity and the Earth. Humans have brought Earth to no more than a composted system of waste. When I asked this question, I thought I would get some special breathing technique for meditation. When I heard the tale of the worm (to be told in the next paragraph), I was amazed at the profundity and wisdom of, not only the story, but the knowing that the survivors must relearn how to breathe the wild of nature into their lives!

The reference to a composted system is creating the analogy of worms that must recycle manure and waste in order to create rich, fertile soil for new growth. If and when there is destruction, humanity will have to reimagine and breathe in nature for renewal. (This particular dialogue was at the end of 2014 and destruction was still a far-fetched idea … I thought. But now it is 2021 and the environment is rapidly declining.)

the airs in the breathing is the same form as this; it's working through the waste or the composite of that which is the man's world. It is looking for that which is the nutrient-rich way of being. The only way it can find the nutrient-rich way of being is to be among the wild of itself. It is wildly looking for that which it has been made from. That which is made for it. That which is conditioned in a way to condition it, as it conditions the composite that it works through.

Language you can use to teach people this breathing would be of sensing their own wild nature. Give them the image of what would you feel like if nothing raised you. All that was in front of you was there to supply you with what you need, and you learn to survive on your own from the beginning of being an infant. You found how to suckle something that was provided for you. After the suckling period you found that which you could put into your mouth and start chewing on, and it would provide nourishment for you and help teeth you as your teeth came through; you stumbled around and found something to chew on and it nourished you further. You chewed on it, you enjoyed it.

Everything you explored from the moment of your infancy was always that which was provided for you, as you discovered it. You found in you that you were the way of you, and the making of you. The only thing you feared, above all else, was this unending feeling of nothing else is like you.

Each step of your search, trying to consume and satisfy this hunger, you find there is nothing like you. You are this strange alien. You never developed a way of speaking. You just mimic the sounds of the birds, the frogs, the howls of the wolves, and the screeching of the owls.

You are overly conditioned to feed what is your immediate need. You never learn to satisfy the need of your aloneness from all that you have experienced outside of you. Finally discovering what is within you, is that which can talk to you … becoming your only friend … that which is inside of you. The voice of God within you.

As you tell your students this story of the wild, they were born a child of the wild, and they discover the only satisfaction they can find in any presence is their own being, a listening to their inner way. That inner way is not affected by the outer way. That inner way is there, no matter what.

You tell people to breathe into this, knowing that they will find God. They will hear the first whispers of God.[138]

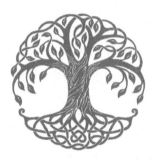

---

138 "Everything that is working you, is what you are working through." This sentence from the above story so succinctly summarizes the heroic process in life of seeking to find God within. It is a testament and a critical process for future generations to re-enliven their "nature-knowing" in order to heal themselves and Earth. The breathing of the airs of the wild is referencing the destruction that is before humankind (unless we wake up) and it is through the imagining of wholeness within that we will find renewal. The other important reference is to information that will be revealed in the next several sessions about how to literally breathe spirit from out of the infinite void into creative manifestation.

SESSION 20

The Will of the Mind

Gary: One of the sessions talked about impressing the body. Is that done by calling the Christ light into the body and bringing in the mind of God to see and feel a new level of awakening?

SOURCE: *Yes. There are conditions for awakening the body you are starting to recognize. The body responds to light coming in from the inner way, by conditioning the parts of it that can get trapped. The focus here is going to be on the mind in the body. The mind isn't something that sits and waits for something to trigger it. The mind is in a constant state of moving. The body can go to moments of rest because it is not an eternal thing. Since it's not eternal, it has moments of rest as a natural part of its function, a natural part of its non-function, a natural part of its in-function.*

An in-function is the programming. In the programming of the body, there are moments of rest, moments of complete rest, and then moments of arrest. In the moments of arrest the body is moving in response to the will of the mind.

The will of the mind in a constant state of movement in a body that has resting periods can get trapped; the mind and the will can get trapped in the sedentary parts of the body. The ego mind can be the resistance that continues on, even as the body incorporates spirit into it. The resistance that resists spirit is the part of the body that is unnoticed, always unnoticed. This resistance is the tenacity of your body's need to be constantly alert where spirit is not alerted in the body.[139]

Gary: The pain that has been mostly unbearable has been the neck and the shoulder. It feels like the pain is seeking to open up a pathway to create a union between mind and heart. Of course, that's the divine mind that feels more and more like it knows that the body is within the mind. As I hold my mind focused and see and feel the light of spirit, the light of Christ moving within, the Eoma is gently beginning to take that form more and more. Sometimes there is a true feeling of light living radiantly and dynamically within.[140]

---

139   The technique I used prior to these sessions was identifying the negative emotion stuck in the body and allowing the light of the Soul to inspire love and healing there. This new teaching was focused on the programs of the ego mind, which can hold deep unconscious beliefs. Down through the centuries humans have been programmed with all kinds of limited concepts and ideas that are contrary to the living-light of spirit entering fully into the body and creating wholeness. These must be ferreted out and released to incorporate Divine Mind in the Christing. As I began this high frequency work of the Christening, I found new areas of the body that were not vibrationally compatible. I experienced some discomfort as I continually upgraded the body to light-body activation. When I began to teach these techniques in my retreats, students would often need to rest a day or two after the retreat, due to the discomfort from restructuring.

140   An important distinction here between Divine mind and ego mind. Divine mind is the mind of the Greater being you are, and a subset of God mind. Your Higher mind has been orchestrating the entire process throughout time/space to master the three-dimensional worlds of form, so that Divine Mind; i.e., God (you are) can live within form.

SOURCE: *It's a physiological conditioning for your body that is related to the Christing manner. Christing, that you call the golden light moving through your body, the Christing has a conscious condition. Golden Light has an effervescent nature to it that is the reflection of the Source from which it comes. The Christing, however, is the taking of that and turning it into an organized being so that it is infused into the body's effervescent manner.*[141]

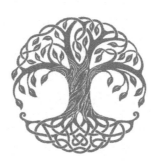

---

141 An individual who steps onto the path of the Great way must Christ themselves. This is accomplished by organizing the Divine mind, along with the feeling nature, into the calling of the Eoma into the body. The Christ organizes the Eoma by holding focused attention upon the images and patterns of wholeness which already exist within the mind of Source/God. They are infused within to create the effervescent light-radiant body of the Christ. This infusion of light is actually the letting go of limiting beliefs; your Soul is already perfect and divine. This is the revelation (revealing) of your true nature.

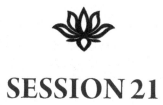

SESSION 21

Sailing With Spirit

SOURCE: *We would like you to know the life you are pursuing is bigger than any life you have pursued thus far, so it's perfectly normal for you to feel small in comparison to the glimpses you're getting. Even though you occasionally feel small compared to the size of this mission, you are not the one who is actually making all of this work. You are the vessel that is showing up so the work can be done. Your smallness only serves to recognize that, and not to put you in a place of feeling less than or in abundance of. Just show up and that's all that's necessary.*[142]

The calling of the Christ will continue to be your teaching's central focus. It is a calling of the Christ for all who live within the vicinity of the call. Even though there may be a small showing of individuals at any given time, the sound will move way beyond the room you are in. People will pick up the feeling from the way they sensitize themselves. Most people have a protective barrier between the world and themselves. Within that protective barrier, this new feeling becomes a

---

142   I was daunted by the scope of the work and wondered if it was possible. Six years later now, I hold to the possibility more clearly as I continue to work tirelessly to embody this profound teaching. And yet, I still humbly understand the greatness of what it fully entails and implies.

marching order that echoes within the chamber of their minds. The echo of the chamber within their minds is the part of them that hears what you are calling them for.

Your message is growing rapidly, not just through the vibration of what you're teaching, but also as you get clearer on the concepts and you become more profound in your own awareness. That profoundation is a flying condition; it flies beyond what is the kite string. So, imagine a kite in flight, connected to the ground by the one that flies the kite; if you clip the string the kite loses its ability to fly until the kite is reassembled in the form of a sail. A sail is connected to a vessel that moves. The kite moves into the system of the vesseling manner and becomes a sail. And you become the captain of that sailing ship.

As you maintain the kite for the time being, you see the kite getting higher and higher, losing tension on the string, making it harder for you to maneuver the ways of the kite. Sometimes it feels out of control. That's when you need to see yourself as the captain of a vessel rather than one who holds onto a string. As you set sail, the mighty vessel that you are captaining has all-hands-on deck, because the storm that doth come forth is a storm that is your entering manner. As you enter into the storm, the sail must come down, the storming seas given over to face what's on the other side of the storm, which is a bright new picture.[143]

---

143   My intuition and feeling during this time of my instruction into the Christing system was that when I achieve a level of radiance, that will be the vibration that emanates out into the world and the appropriate people will respond to it. At the same time, there were frequent gifts in the dialogues to encourage me, and analogies to help me see how beautifully the work was progressing, such as … sailing through the stormy seas to the bright new picture!

Gary: Is there anything I am doing that disrupts my purpose?

SOURCE: *You are doing everything that is in line with the mission. Is there anything you're doing that disrupts your sense of obligation to the mission? Yes. There are times that you are in a forgetful mode about your own importance. You forget how important you are, and that forgetting needs to be mitigated with moments of remembering the historical truth of it all. Historical truth must be forwarded in every generation to the next one. The profound condition of each generation is about the investment of the work. For instance, Rumi was never as popular as he is now. That's the legacy of the work. There are people who have made their legacy profound in the time of their living. Mary Baker Eddy was one of them, which is why she was chosen to be your guide. But the scope of it can be so burdensome for you at times that you forget the importance of it. How do you remember it? Just look at the world and how devastated it is.*[144]

---

144   I have never wavered from the path. But I also know the importance of this work is so much greater today than it was only 7 years ago when this dialogue took place. Political turmoil, financial disparity, hunger, disease, and maybe the most disruptive, the technology that traps so many young minds in their small screens of videos and social media, are all part and parcel of the environmental collapse plaguing the Earth, and thereby, humanity.

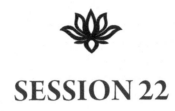

SESSION 22

Light Emanation

Gary: It feels like the void is an open doorway within the heart, and arising out of it are infinite possibilities of God becoming. (Sondra had the image of a spider weaving its web).

SOURCE: *This opening within you, Gary, is the portal to the void. In that portal, you become your own journey system. It's in this system that the void can never understand its own Nature, because it journeys itself over and over again, looking for a reflection of that which is its worth. When its worth is something that has no value to spirit, it becomes an enclosed, encased, and incarcerated form of existence that all too many people live. When you understand your value and worth to spirit, your journey becomes expansive and no longer has boundaries of three-dimensional form. It's in this expansive reach that Sondra experienced as the spider. God as the spider in the void ... the ever-expanding reach that is the arms of the spider, the reach.*[145]

---

145   Within the void the unmanifest possibilities of Source/God hover within the "no-thing." Spirit swirls within the darkness knowing not that which it is, looking for a reflection. When an individual brings light into the darkness, through the light of the Christ System, they become their own journey system of expansion. The expression of their creative joy, within infinite possibilities, is symbolic of the spider weaving its web of creation from out of the velvety nighttime into the light of knowing.

Gary: Yes, many thousands of tendrils of the void reaching out to purpose itself. It is from out of the open doorway that we can breathe those possibilities, through the lens of the Christ, and create more of God seeing God's self.

SOURCE: *Yes, God seeing what God can be.*

Sondra: Where is the Christ energy related to this picture of the void of the spider?

SOURCE: *The spider reaching into itself and recognizing that within itself is the power of its own making. The void knowing within itself, a higher abundance of itself. Recognizing that it is only in the acknowledgement of itself that it can be a Christed energy.*[146]

Sondra: The void is not conscious of its own consciousness?

SOURCE: *Correct. The void is not conscious of its own consciousness. However, when the Christing becomes accessible to the consciousness that is not conscious of itself, the reflection of itself in the Christ-light acknowledges the further reaches of the self-enjoyment. The Christ strumming light.*[147]

Sondra: The vibration, the music, sound?

---

146   Like a spider spinning its crystalline web from inside out, the crystalline light of the Christ illuminates what God could be within the void and summons it into manifestation through the Eoma. The Eoma is the sparkling effervesce that twinkles these illuminated holograms into visible form.

147   Creation originated as sound vibration, transforming to become light activation, in order for Source to express itself into form to see what IT might be. This unconditional birthing and giving is the highest expression of love. The universe is a manifestation of love, and equally significant, you came from … and are part of … this creator being of love.

SOURCE: *Yes. Imagine the void as its own expansive land; it's an existence in and of itself. All that exists, exists within the void. But if the void is not conscious of itself, it knows not the thing that it is not. It knows not that you are not the void. It just imagines you as being what it is.*

Sondra: When I recognize myself in an organized manner as an organized physical being here, the void is not seeing you this way.

SOURCE: *Right, it cannot see. It cannot hear, it cannot feel, it cannot sense at all.*

Sondra: So, I'm a Christed manifestation of the void?

SOURCE: *Yes, you are a Christed manifestation of the void, thereby giving light to that which has worth. Whereas the void is a way of existence that cannot reflect upon itself.*

Gary: Yes, darkness can't reflect darkness. It has to have light to reflect it, to mirror it.

SOURCE: *Yes, the void wanting to know itself creates that which it can reflect upon.*

Sondra: Oh, so that's the Christing?

SOURCE: *That's the Christing. It is the void <u>yearning</u> to know itself, so it expands within itself in a continual annihilation of the dark.*[148]

Sondra: Are those the new stars being birthed in the star nurseries, which are composed of galactic dust?

SOURCE: *Correct, one after another, like a pulse in a living breathing being.*

---

148   The Christ system (light) arose from the yearning of spirit within the void to know itself; to bring illumination into the darkness. The Christing is the prismatic formulation of light into physicality in-order for Source to know its "worth". The yearning of Source to know itself posited the question, "What Am I?" And there was light!

Gary: Now that I opened the portal into the void, I can create (symbolic) stars of creation?

SOURCE: *Absolutely.*[149]

Sondra: How radiant can that light emanation be?

Gary: I think it depends upon how focused one's consciousness is, and how you are able to call forth spirit as the power. With dynamic focus and love, you could feel it coming through the Christed lens with dynamic radiance. It would also depend upon how long you could hold the focus and clarity that would be needed to create the size and the magnitude of the "starburst."

Sondra: God, is this what Gary is going to create with his students in the workshops?

SOURCE: *We haven't fully described that, and we aren't ready to divulge this because each individual must believe they are creating it. However, the light coming up in the room is Gary's worthying what he has described. The more worthying that goes inward to this knowing that your ability is to project this light from the void, the more you will know the Christ. It's a vibration of light activated by the being that knows itself as a condition of the void moving through the higher ether and praising that which is in the room.*

---

149   This is a beautiful image of Source/God birthing "itself" from out of the void into the great star systems. A newborn star gathers the dust of the universe (Eoma) and creates planets to purpose its life. The planets create life to reflect their possibilities in materiality, and then spirit, which began creation, enters into materiality as consciousness, and God awakens on Earth; i.e., into materiality. Then, most exquisitely, the human can Christ themselves and summon from the void new possibilities; further expanding the always becoming nature of Source.

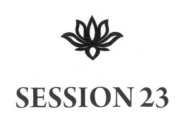

SESSION 23

Radiance

Gary: When I meditate it feels like an opening here (gesturing to the heart chakra) that is a hollow place inside of me. When I meditate it becomes an entry point into the void that is quite profound. It feels like the breath of spirit is erupting. Then it begins to work on my body through my neck and the upper body quadrant. Is there something I am doing in error?[150]

SOURCE: *What you're experiencing is the fireball. The fireball can create problems for the body if it doesn't have a good sire. The sire is always about reproduction in the exact condition as that which is reproducing itself; it's a siring.*

In the siring for you, that means you need to imagine the ripple effect of light from you into the world. Not into the earth in the way that you ground yourself, but rather the siring that is the expansion into world. You can do it by creating a new imagination the minute it starts to feel as if there is an abundance of anacartion.

---

150   The transformation of the gross physical body into a higher dimensional form means that all the cells, tissues, bones, blood, and nerves must go through an upgrade in vibration. I was so dedicated and focused in my meditations (as well as doing workshops and counseling), that several times I experienced a great deal of discomfort in the body. After these transformations, which could take several weeks or even a month to heal, I then experienced a new level of consciousness in the body. I also think this level of discomfort would be rare for most individuals on the path because I was being directed to create light activation within in order to activate light around.

The anacartion is when the body experiences what is meditation incarnate. It is ana-cartion, ana—meaning all, and cartion—meaning carnate. All oneness in the body. It's an all oneness that is too much for the body so that all "oneness" needs to expand into the world. You are going into the world; the anacartion is a ripple into the foundations of that which is your expansion. You expand into the world that which is from the void; the fire in the way of your Christing condition. As that fire expands, it expands into the echolection.[151]

---

151   For thirty-five years prior to my work with Source, I taught grounding, to stabilize the body with the Earth, so I could be conscious of all seven chakras in order to clear them of negative emotion. I facilitated hundreds of aura readings, and I was able to discern that most individuals (even those on a high spiritual path), had little or no light below the diaphragm. This problematic area included the 3rd chakra of self-empowerment at the navel, the 2nd chakra of emotion and feeling in the pelvic region, and the 1st chakra at the base of the spine for grounding. When you can identify the negative emotion in the body without judgment (not examining it with the mind but feeling it with the heart), you can symbolically slip through the dark emotion and begin to love yourself at the physical and emotional levels. This release allows the greater knowing within the Higher mind to be activated and embodied. You no longer know the truth; you embody the truth.

I taught this emotional clearing process in my earlier workshops. In meditation, the student would open their crown chakra at the top of the head and see/feel golden light flowing down completely in and through the body. The next instruction was to open the base of the spine chakra and imagine golden streamers of light flowing in and through Mother Earth, which grounded the physical body and allowed the student to feel where dark emotion was still stuck in the body. This might take five or ten minutes to discern. The next step was to see/feel the light of the Higher self or Soul moving into that area in order to embrace the emotion with unconditional love. The Soulful feeling of Self-love allowed the emotion to be released, and over time effected the healing of all seven chakras. This had been my personal process, which allowed me to heal and balance a difficult childhood and release the corresponding negative emotions stored in the tissues and organs. This prepared me for what, I was to learn in these sessions, was the Christing system. Source recognized this and was now having me switch gears into a higher order of light activation. With this new technique I was focusing the awakened fireball of light from within, rippling it out into the world.

When you're with your students, they are the echolection. You expand the expression of you into them. They hold it so you aren't holding it alone. You give it a direction, a course and an embodiment. Then your embodiment is expanded by the number of people in the room that you're expanding it to. This is why you are going into silence as you teach. The silence is that expansion of the anacartion into the echolection.

As anacartion expands, you have less demand on your body, more of a command on the other bodies. This is what requires silence in your meditation in this system of many. If you were to continue to speak the way you do, you would cause more internal radiation damage. We've been waiting for you to take this question into your own mind, which you've done. In that question you've expanded your body's condition. This expansion then causes you no way out, so now you're forced to ask the question verbally. With that verbal question we describe what you're experiencing; you just don't know you're experiencing it. You don't know that what you're experiencing is a literal form of your expansion. You have imagined it as being more like a figurative form of your expansion, but it is literal, and you begin to expand into the very people who will acknowledge this in a very complex way.[152]

---

152   One of the dynamic aspects of the Christing is the alleviation or letting go of our personality constructs. We realize that the Higher mind creates the body and holds it within a molecular suspension. This allows the Christ system to illuminate beyond the body and creates the fireball of light that can ignite others. This is called a transmission of energy rather than a teaching. I was being instructed about how to enter deeper into the silence to affect this process.

Sondra: I just got a flash. This is how ascended masters work when they're in spirit, how Jesus can have a relationship with millions of people or Mother Mary or any of the ascended masters. The practice of anacartion is going to go beyond the passing of your physical body, Gary. Is that right, God?

SOURCE: *Yes, this is how this works. This is how you create a following and how this following expands beyond your death. Your mastery rises-up into the etheric aura, the omnipresence; this is creating omnipresence. The omnipresence you create in silence will be the repetition of silence. Silence in this manner isn't just not speaking, silence is an array; you create an array of you. The one of you creates new ones of you. Each new one of you creates more ones of you. This is the rippling effect of the firing condition … a firing up. It fires up the spirit in each individual, and as that fire up occurs, they get louder in spirit and you see it. You see the dynamic condition of it in each of their bodies as you are systematically expressing it. It's not just an experience, it's an expression experience.*

Ex-perience is the key word we want you to recall when you feel this hot flame of fire. Recall ex-perience and you travel with the experience in the expression. We want you to imagine this now. [153]

Sondra: Like a candle lighting other candles. It keeps lighting, getting more and more aflame.

---

153   This is the essence of "transmission teaching;" you are expressing the living light into another's body and igniting their divine presence. In spirit words it is referred to as "explace" light.

SOURCE: *Correct. It doesn't remove the flame from the candle, it multiplies the flame. When you're alone (and not in a group that can "explace" you and enable you as it expands the body of you to all those that are there, just as light increases by the amount of lights that are lit), you <u>imagine</u> all the others lighting up; that's what you will be doing. This way, you're not carrying all the light because grounding doesn't work to save you from it. Grounding just makes it actually more pronounced. Grounding is counter to what you've trained yourself for thirty five years. Now you know what to do.*[154]

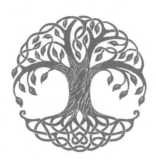

---

154   When consciousness awakens into a higher dimensional knowing, it transcends beyond the three-dimensional construct of time and space. This can be a concept hard to grasp until you experience it. In this condition, the imagination draws the desired image/ person into focus and the Eoma precipitates light-matter around them. Transmission is then possible from a distance as you see and feel the imaged person in wholeness, love and light. There have been many recorded instances of healing at a distance (sometimes through prayer) and this is a similar concept.

SESSION 24

Power of the Pyramid

Gary: In our first reading you talked about an organization I would create.

SOURCE: *The Gary Springfield is going to be an organization of its own and will have an effect on those who live beyond Gary Springfield's time on the Earth.*

The Springfield is a condition of the field of the abundance, the abundance field. This abundance field is a wide net that is cast across four generations. These generations are not just mother to son and son to daughter. These are generations of individuals who already know you and who will be sharing the information they are trained in by you. The condition of this training is mindfulness training and you call it the Golden Light system.

When one incorporates an understanding of the nature of the Golden Light, what is one learning about oneself? When one becomes the Golden Light, when one is iridescent in the Golden Light, what is "one" in this Golden Light? One is a system of true being. When one is iridescent in the Golden Light, one is true being. The true being is a nature that is individual and perfect. It is <u>perfected before</u> the individual acknowledges it is perfected. Identifying individual perfection is the nature of the most way of the individual perceptualizing one's *own distance.*[155]

Hold onto this because it's not something that is clear to you in the evidence, meaning there is no evidence that's going to show you this is true. It can only come from an experience of your faith pulling through what is the knowing of you from what has already been before the body was born. This body is a vessel that has to constantly be refreshed in its in-tranced state. It is your meditations that refresh you. Every refreshing is a reigniting of this nature. Every reigniting of this nature is a calling forth of it to you, and as it calls to you, you remember it. As you remember it, you become it over and over again.[156]

This is the life of the transition. You were never meant to be in a state of being. The state of being is something that you have to remember as you "enayorate" your layers. An enayorating occurs when there is a natural identity. It is a nayer patience. A natural identity is a nayer patience. The nayer patience is a condition of remembering the body is not what you are. Every time you remember this, the intergalactic nature of you starts to remember the transition this body really is. This body is not an implant into the world, it is a transitional state of three dimensions for your higher way.

In the identity of your Higher-being, you will get to watch what unfolded as a result of this enayorbation; it's an enayorbation of this body. It is the movement of your being that envelops the condition of three dimensions, then moves back into its wave. In this short time on the planet you will have done something for the planet. The nature of this empire will grow. It's been seeded. You have seeded

---

155   When an individual becomes iridescent in the Golden Light one has systematized their true being. The true being is already perfect and the task is to perceptualize it … image-in this truth and acknowledgment it within form.

156   The greater being I AM was preconditioned with the full knowing of the mission for this lifetime. As I pull that awareness in and through via meditation (over and over again) I become it; i.e., the evidence of this will be made manifest through the actualization in the body.

it in the field of spring.[157] (Enayorbation is a Spirit word.)

Gary: You mentioned in one of our sessions that life on the Earth is affiliated with the Galactic Federation. What is that?

SOURCE: *As you revel in the thought that you've created a seed on the planet, we get to tell you both something quite magnificent. The Galactic empire is one that has extended way beyond the surface of this planet. It is a galactic condition that is way older than life on this planet. It goes into the life of other planets, and it hovers and hovers. It is a hovering condition that identifies when a planet is ready for full life abundance. In this manner, the condition is not just in an individual, it's in an entire team of individuals. There are teams of individuals who come to this planet at the same time in order to bring the wave (that is led by certain individuals) forward. Some individuals in the wave are there supporting the wave and some are leading the wave. Every wave that is led out is a wave that has come at a specific time in the history of humankind, not in the history of the individual, the history of the human.*[158]

The next station in this development is to be in communication. Communication in the way of spirit are crystalline formations. These crystalline formations create prisms of light, prisms of attribution and prisms of reflection. These

---

157 I was familiar with the concept of the Soul pre-conditioning itself in each lifetime to play out its role in physicality. Here it's being said that my current incarnation is a movement of my Higher being into the wave of this three-dimensional lifetime to perform a function. As I, Gary Springfield, continue to remember that I am not this body and accomplish my mission, I will one day remember, in spirit, the Field of Spring that was seeded by this information. So, the nature of the community grows on Earth in the Spring-Field of the Christening.

158 This concept of a Federation of enlightened beings from many star systems seeding planets that were ready for life was not a new concept to me. I was aware that over the time-line of human history there were several star groups that worked with evolving humanity. Some say alien influences were parenting an evolving species, while other extra-terrestrials were quite domineering, manipulative and controlling.

are the arrays, and those arrays must be set in place.

The One Hundred is the main array to be assembled, but each stage of that is as important as the previous stage. The first stage that's been assembled is the founding condition. The next stage of the condition is going to be that which responds to the foundation. We're working on that now.[159]

Sondra: So this is a war?

SOURCE: *Yes. This is a war that will be embattling some of the worst and darkest natures of human-kind. It's in that embattlement that the opinion of the winners will be formed. The winners have to be opinioned, and they cannot be opinioned when they feel themselves unable to fight for anything important. You have to give them something to fight for. What they are fighting for is the light. And they are fighting for the way of God. The way of God evermore away from tyranny. As tyranny grows, which we promise you will see soon, tyranny is already in its alignment and ready to zoom.*

There are already conditions of accomplishment that are losing ground in the light. Not that we would allow that for very long, just long enough for people to see how important their alignment to the light is. No longer can they ignore or be apathetic to that which is growing in the dark. That which grows in the dark grows evermore; it never stops. As we expose the light to it, it ceases to grow. So we expose light over and over again. Expose light. Overcoming the darkness means that all light must explode into its own nature … always revealing the light!

This is a system of the evermore. It is the system of the growing way and the system of the knowing way. Each consciousness must align to this or it cannot be

---

159   It was interesting to hear those communications on the higher order are crystalline formations, which makes sense, when we now use fiber optics to carry information. This could give a hint to a future technology on the planet. (The foundation referenced above was established in the reading of the One Hundred in Session Five.)

conscious on the planet, and the dying of the planet will occur. All dying of the planet is in the acknowledgement of darkness. It's only in the acknowledgement of the light that it can grow to the brighter way, and the knowing of the light is the knowing of the growing of the way. Each growing of the way is an acknowledgement of its own tenacity to be. Tenacity to be is the light of the being that is in all things, and all things that are in tune with this accrue in light.

As darkness starts to reveal itself on the planet through the human mind, the human mind must go into war, and the war that it becomes is the war of darkness engulfing Earth. Believe you me, this is not what the human wants to see. So every human must be informed in light or it will create a dark, dark night. Each dark night is the source of all corridors. That corridor feeds on itself. It feeds on itself until there is no light that can even penetrate it.[160]

Sondra: What's the purpose of the darkness destroying the light?

SOURCE: *Power. Great power. Power that is in its own single right. The power that can destroy all things of light. This is a power so profound that even God shakes when it comes near. Not because it destroys God, but because it destroys all that God makes. When it destroys all that God makes, God watches what God makes being destroyed. Even that can cause destruction.*

It's only in the reminder of what God is, over and over again in the making, always creating, always giving, always releasing, always an expression, always

---

160   It did not surprise me that this was spoken of as a war. I heard there was an intergalactic war on the higher dimensions between the forces of the dark and the light, and it was a fight to hold this planet in its foundation of Christ, in order to secure the evolution of humanity and Earth. But humanity has slipped into a pattern of ignorance as money, power, glamour, and consumerism have brought the planet to a place of ecological disaster. This book is preparing humanity, if there is devastation, to know the self-actualizing nature of the Christing, and to create a new world; symbolically, the heaven on Earth of peace and plenty. As one passage said in Session Five, "We don't fear that the destruction is happening, we are watching it." This information is the preparation for those who would choose to grow into the light.

a giving way. When God is reminded of that giving way, then God does not see that which is the destroying way. The giving way is the light of the All way. The All way becomes the evermore. In the evermore, all are free. All are free.[161]

⚘ ⚘ ⚘

Gary's Questions:

Gary: How does one understand Christ consciousness in the symbol of the Egyptian pyramids?

SOURCE: *We would like to adjust your question to the nature of the pyramid itself. Put yourself in the middle of that pyramid. Look up into the capstone. When you put yourself there, in the center of that pyramid and you look up into the capstone, what do you experience?*

Gary: The exaltation of the spirit above.

SOURCE: *Correct. Now look at it physics-wise. Look at the geometrical form that you're creating in the center of that. When energy is coming from all points, and you are in the center of that. What's happening to you? What are the points actually doing as they meet in you? What are they doing to you?*

---

161   The darkness is the power grasping, controlling, manipulating forces on a cosmic level, as well upon the Earthly realm. This destroys love and light. The giving way, and the way of light and love are the true foundation of creation that bestows freedom on all beings to make their own way. Earth is at an evolutionary crossroad and people must awaken to the internal knowing of God within, the foundation of all life. Religion still posits an external God that will save us if we repent, pray and give them our money and power. In times past, it's possible that religion did play a part in the development of humanity, but now we must awaken and summon the One Source within all.

Gary: The divine effulgence, it starts to ignite?

SOURCE: *There is ignition, and in that ignition there's really an energy ball that's being generated. It's a ball of light and it's floating you. It's keeping you in a state of suspension. It is coming into the center of you from all points of the pyramid. You become the golden being in the center. It is a golden being because from the top of the capstone is the source light from the top into the crown of the head. Meeting you there are the four points that are at the bottom of the pyramid, which create in the center of you an entirely new capstone. You become another capstone, replicating the condition of the Source capstone from the above.*

You become a trigger, you become a selective form of adjustment. You can adjust at any point which way to move from the center. You are a floating being, held in suspension.

Sondra (drawing on paper): So here you're in this center and there is a beam that goes into your crown from above, and a beam from each corner going into you. You are about one third of the way up in the center of the pyramid.

Gary: Does the energy ignite and go up like a laser going up out of the cap?

SOURCE: *No, think of yourself as not the ignited one, but the igniting one. You are drawing from these corners, drawing from each point. As you draw all that within, that light is electrically building in you. It's all points being drawn into you igniting and it is collectively building at your center. As this collection is building, this is you drawing which is the nature of the Christ.*

This is the calling. The calling, the drawing to you, the acknowledging of you to the you. This is you making the God-Self. You call to the Christ and the Christ to you. You build the Christed energy that comes from the Eoma. It's only in the calling of that, and the calling to that, which creates the Christed tenacity. As you call God, God calls you.[162]

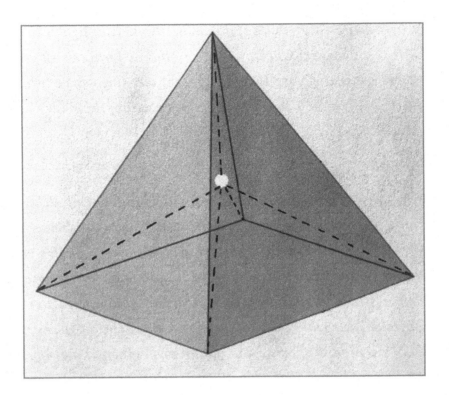

$\mathcal{T}$he Pyramid is the structure of power. At the interior center there is the "calling" to Source. The five interior points emanate electric-blue energy that intersects in the middle, awakening the individual Mind of God within the "One Calling". The Breath of Spirit arising from the void creates life.

---

162   In prior sessions there had been hints about how one could understand the Christ system though the pyramids. This clear explanation of the creation and ignition of an electrified ball of energy, created by "calling" the five points to the center of the pyramid, proved to be a dynamic powering-up in my light activation. The created ball Is the electric blue field of Divine mind, and in the center of that is the golden Christ star. This is the divine assembly of light that manifests the Christ and opens the interior doorway within the heart, back into the realms of spirit/void. This is the essence of the Christing.

Sondra: Why do I see a blue light in this?

SOURCE: *The blue light is the God light. The Christ light is the golden light. The golden light is to create a sense of acclimatization. Blue light is to call forth that which is the highest condition of the crystalline form, which really does nothing except ignite the way. The golden light can then move through that ignited way. The blue light is the process of the structure; the golden light is the process of the being.*

Sondra: Is either one more beneficial than another in any given situation?

SOURCE: *Yes, the golden light is beneficial for any state of being. Whenever you are in a state of disassembly, calling upon the golden light to relieve you of that disassembly will give you a sense of peace in any situation, relieving you of any stress, relieving you of any assimilation. Also, to assimilate to other people's way of being, you present to them the golden light you are, and you will be relieved of assimilating to anything other than what is your way of being. In your own way of being there is a process of peace and in that peace, there is a giving to others what is their way of being. The golden light is being. The condition of the blue light is highly beneficial when you want to retrieve the imagination of the way of God for you. So, grow into the blue light in order to see past the initial way. The initial way is what's happening right now. When you want to see what is in the past or in the future, but in a way that is beneficial to the right now, open up the blue light. The blue light carries information. Golden light is information. Blue light carries it.*[163]

---

163   Blue light is the high frequency of Source light and carries information embedded within it. In order to know things, you enter into that light. Golden light is organic living-light, because it is an emanation of the Christ system, which is the creative mechanism of life.

Gary: Would it be beneficial to imagine the pyramid structure around you and then draw energy from it?

SOURCE: *Absolutely. We recommend you teach it so that it illustrates an individual's way in their sitting position. If they can see themselves sitting in the center of the pyramid, then they can slowly start to feel what is the way of this in being it. Putting yourself in the center of that without seeing the self ... but being the self in the imagined way. That's the goal.*[164]

Gary: In the past there have been times when my body has been achy regardless of what I eat or how I sleep. Growing pains or assimilating energy?

SOURCE: *When consciousness is high, the cells in the body separate a bit so there is space for the flow. When consciousness is low, it slams back together and aches. Those cells no longer have that space, they densify and ache. There's no way to avoid it and there is no way to remove yourself from that experience. You have to manage your level of pain, and you can do that through pain mitigation if you feel the necessity.*[165]

---

164   Oftentimes when people imagine, they create an external image of themselves and place that image in the pyramid. Here, it is being instructed for the individual to feel themselves there, and then look out through their eyes and imagine the pyramid structure all around. Then see/feel the call of energy from the five points for their ignition and self-actualization.

165   Over time, I found the cells become less resistant to this phenomenon as the vibrational tone of the body increases in synchronization with spirit. Until then, an aspirin or two every now and again was helpful.

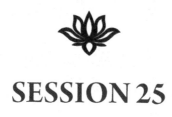

SESSION 25

Summoning Source

Gary: We were talking about the pyramid and how the pyramid is the structure that ignites the Christ. Isn't it a star tetrahedron?

SOURCE: *The pyramid is not that structure. The pyramid is a square and triangle configuration. This square and triangle configuration is the structure of creation. There are four and three, four and three. You, as the center being, become the created being.*

Sondra: Source is at the capstone … and then from the four corners?

SOURCE: *Which is also Source. From the four corners is also Source.*[166]

Sondra: What's the Christed nature?

SOURCE: *The Christed nature is the being that is calling. Calling Source from the source of the power structure of this pyramid. So, too, in the Christed way there is a calling from Source. Calling from Source, to Source, for Source, by Source, of Source, with Source. We aren't sure you recognize the power in this. The power of it is a play on words.*

166   Source is summoned to the center way by your "calling" of the energy-points in the pyramid to meet there. This ignites the being who is "calling" the Source of power to them. Similarly, within the great pyramid of Egypt there are chambers within the interior that were probably used in initiation ceremonies to evolve life.

Sondra: The power of it is a play on words. You mean that this construction or this structure that's created is a power source?

SOURCE: *Yes, a power source.*

Gary: Isn't it from the star tetrahedron that the flower of life is created, which is also one of the matrixes of God's creation?

SOURCE: *Yes, but it's not the same structure. It's a completely different structure than the pyramid. The Christed way is a structure of individual power, the structure of the creative condition; that is the flower of life and it's the giving way. And that is a giving way that is an evermore. It's evermore. It cannot be created because it is what it is. It just <u>is</u> creating. It is the verb form of the condition. The pyramid condition is a noun. It is an existence that is made, not an existence that is eternal. If it were eternal there could be no creation in organic power. Organic power is something so much gentler and softer. It can be quickly destroyed by the power that is generated through the calling of power from Source if it is abused.*

Pure Source is a power structure. The Christing is a calling of that power structure. The Christing is used for manipulating the Eoma as an organizing system. It's an organizing power structure. When it's misused, it's used as a way of tyranny. It's a way of organizing all that is the structuring of a people. And when you turn that structure in on itself, it becomes its own burden.[167]

---

167   On the path of awakening an individual begins to imagine and feel the Christ energy within. Over time, awareness flowers and leads to the realization of the pyramid structure, which becomes a conscious calling from Source to ignite the way. The awakened Christ calls to the power of Source, summoning spirit from the field of all possibilities, in order to inform life.

Sondra: Like a beast of burden?

SOURCE: *Yes. Human populations can be made into beasts of burden through this power structure.*[168]

The flower of life is the power structure of Mother Nature giving. The misuse of power is the condition that Moses experienced. The Egyptians used the power source to evoke pure domination. This same structure can also be used to override a dominant structure. It is power upon power. It is power for freedom, power freeing, that Moses used.

Sondra: Moses called to Source and used the Christed way to organize his people out of Egypt?

SOURCE: *Yes indeed.*[169]

Gary: In meditation this morning, I created a pyramid. I sat in the center of it and a golden fiery sun began to develop that was phenomenal.

SOURCE: *We would like to know where in your mastery do you feel the biggest shift as a result of what you created? There has been a significant shift.*

Gary: Two things. One is calling Source from the void (from within). Two is calling the electric blue light from the apex and the corners of the pyramid. The electric blue ignited the sunlit Christ energy and in the center of that is the void. Around the void is the ignited sunlight of the Christ; i.e., sun/son energy within the pyramid.

---

168   When the power structure is used in tyranny, then it is not the Christ that is creating; it is the summoning of power by the ego for personal will. You might call this black magic, and a dark adept or magician can only take themselves to a certain level of manipulating physicality. Whereas, the Christ is One with Source, calling spirit from the void to create life anew.

169   A beautiful example of what I described in the footnote above ... Christ essence is love, life and freedom. Moses summoned the power of Source, and through the Christed way, organized the flight to freedom.

SOURCE: *Yes. Major accomplishment. This is also what Sondra saw. We know she saw it because she was reflecting what you were creating. She's powerful enough to create it on her own, but not disciplined enough. When you were able to create this in her mind's eye, she can now establish the discipline to make it happen. This is what you're going to be doing for others.*

Your students will identify who is in the core of that pyramid. Who is that? What is that? It is the Being of the Self ... the Self as it is related to the Source ... Source as it is related to the Christed way. And what you recognized in that void in the center was the God within, the All within. Not just the "I" thing, but the whole thing, so that the "I" becomes the independent system for which the being perfects the self in the God way.[170]

Sondra: The whole thing is made to identify the I?

SOURCE: *Yes, The I of God within.*

Gary: It becomes a creator God.

SOURCE: *Indeed. All creator God conditions require the human to completely divorce the human condition. There is nothing in the human condition that is remotely like it. You cannot sit down and manipulate material to create something in three-dimensional form that is remotely similar to what is created in the essence of the creator God within. The creator God within can summon an entire ecosystem to begin and end in a mere thought. No human being on the planet is capable of this because it requires a system of alignment that could not support a human body. It is the creator status that assembles righteousness when in the human form, so that all conditions of moving*

---

170   This was my initial awakening and acknowledgment of the sunlit being I Am summoning Source from the void. It was also confirmed that this will be part of the teaching of the Christed way, which I had not been introduced to yet. When the teaching began, the acceleration in my own awareness was like being on a rocket ship; so much joy and magnificence within the Christing experience.

forward are in the righteous way.[171]

Sondra: So that's how big movements are possible.

SOURCE: *Correct. Big movements are not possible without it.*

Sondra: Is that the mirroring effect when each individual is touched by it ... the array?

SOURCE: *No, it's not the array (yet) at that stage. At this stage it's just the mirroring. There is an identity question: Who am I? And in the expression of the who am I, the wondering of the who starts to mirror the horror of human tragedy.*

Sondra: How do they mirror the horror of human tragedy?

SOURCE: *They begin to see that the world is living in a completely created way, and the created way is a horrifying condition. That's the first condition that creates a movement's essential nature. Someone must do something. So they look for that someone who's doing something and they start to align with that. For some people this means shaving their head and joining the Hare Krishnas. For others this means getting involved in politics. Others may simply identify a liberation of their own mind. Each individual who has a structure within the movement can be a part of the movement or a part of their own life alteration.*[172]

---

171   It is beautiful to imagine the magnitude of manifestation possible when one surrenders the human 'I' and gives themselves over to the Christing within. As Jesus said, "All that God is I AM." Source is revealing the step-by-step process.

172   Stepping onto the path and conditioning oneself is done through the process of mirroring. The question: "what am I or what can I be?" looks for its reflection in the world from books, people, experiences, and most importantly, one's own imagination. When the most important question is asked: "What can I imagine I Am?" With time and discipline, it will be so. This is internal mirroring. At the same time, when you reflect upon the travesty occurring in the world, it demands the question: "What will I mirror that is new and grand?" The Christ mirrors Source, and is a creator being of love and freedom for all.

Sondra: When I was picturing the pyramid I was also in the center, and I was picturing myself as this gathering ball of energy. There was a knitting effect of light and energy in this blue ball of light.[173]

SOURCE: *That creates the calling condition. The more you create the calling condition, the more you will manifest what you call.*

Gary: The primary purpose of the pyramid is to enhance the calling within us?

SOURCE: *To bring calling to manifest. It's to "powerize" you.*

Ed F: If we get it without the pyramid, which Gary has been trying to do, it's just harder.

SOURCE: *Correct. As soon as Gary was given this tool, it becomes an accelerator. The only reason he wasn't given this tool sooner is that he wasn't ready to withhold all of that power. He was always giving that power away because he wants everyone to be in the same space of growth. But now that Gary is being surrounded by those who are able to grow with him, he can put himself in a state where he accelerates those around him.[174]*

The people who Gary is invoking are not to power him, he is to power them. It is their calling for their own way of life to begin its process of true evolution that he was called to Earth in the first place. There was a need for someone to teach the way of manifest, someone to teach the Christed way and bring into the Christed way a new dynamic.

---

173   I liked this image of calling to Source as though you were knitting a radiant ball of electric blue light all around you.

174   In the calling, it was reiterated over and over again that it was Source calling to Source for Source, rather than a calling from the personal self. When I imagined myself as Source calling Source, the electrified event took on another level of power and dynamics.

For now, the Christ is Jesus Christ, and that keeps the system too small. The Christed way has to increase in numbers if the planet is to evolve, and if human consciousness is to evolve. We needed someone to come to Earth and diminish the impact of Jesus Christ the myth by giving the Christed way a whole new conversation. It had to be de-sold.[175]

Sondra: You mean the Jesus Christ story has been sold?

SOURCE: *Yes, the original language was lost. The story was lost and language was created to control people.*

Gary: Is there any need for us to know more about the ridge beings or who they are?

SOURCE: *The ridge dwellers are 4th dimensional beings that work with Souls. If they are working with Souls and do not have a beneficial message for humankind, the Souls that get caught up in the messages of the ridge ones are Souls that could be lost. To be clear, it is important to remind people there is only one God. No aliens, no angels, no money, no nothing other than the one God. Check with God before you ever give up your beliefs to someone about anything. Always check with your inner God. If you have no connection to your inner God, find out how. In the future, when people start to worship that which they do not understand because it has more power than they do, they can easily*

---

175   Religious indoctrination proclaimed Jesus as the savior who died for our sins. Christ is not a person, it is the creative field of manifestation that stands at the doorway between spirit and matter, and summons spirit from the void in order to create life. Jesus mastered this system and said; "It is not I, but the Father within me that does the work," meaning spirit arises forth from out of the void to create life. The Christ identifies those possibilities within the void and summons spirit to make them real. He didn't come to save humanity, he came to show them the way of embodying the Christ in order to save themselves and create a heaven on Earth experience for all.

be separated from the nature of their Soul that is connected to God.[176]

Gary: Is any of that connected to the anti-Christ?

SOURCE: *The anti-Christ is simply the condition that supports tyranny. The Christ is the nature of the way that is freedom for all. All are free because all are God, and all are natures of God, free to be. The anti-Christ is that which supports some form of tyranny. There can be tyranny in the body; i.e., tyrannical in a body as in addiction. The body constantly wants and wants more. To keep it from wanting, it is given everything it wants. This is slavery, enslaving the body into some form of addiction. It can also be slavery to extra-terrestrial tyranny. Christing relieves any form of tyranny into freedom. Freedom from tyranny.*

Gary: As we hold ourselves in the Christed way in alignment with God, there's nothing to worry about regarding Annunaki or aliens.

SOURCE: *Exactly. These beings cannot come near the sunlight. They can distract you by doing things that rupture your comfort. They can hide things from you and send people to you that have a destructive message to give you. They can do those things, but so long as you are trained to call upon the Christed way through the way of Source being, then those things have no impact.*

If you told people the effects of the day are being caused by the Annunaki, it could incarcerate the individual in language that is inappropriate. Similar to what they do with astrology; i.e., Mars is in retrograde. They are constantly finding ways to not take responsibility. We recommend you focus on sharing tools to call upon the Christed way when things seem to be in disarray and

---

176   There is only one identity, Source/God, in which you live, move and have your being; an eternal ocean of Oneness. Be the ocean of God's identity, and no-thing of darkness can come unto you.

disorder. It's a way of realigning.[177]

The Annunaki are not ones to draw you into depression. They are ones to distract you from the lighted way. Depression comes from thought. Thought can be impacted by an Annunaki affecting someone else to say something to trigger all of your darkest thoughts, but they cannot physically bring you down. The Christed way is uplifting you ... and isn't uplifting you up and out of something outside of you. If you need uplift, it's because your thoughts are off. The things going on inside of you are not being disciplined, they're being left to run on their own and run amuck.

When you work your meditation in a way that silences the mind, brings in the Christed light, then you are taking all of those thoughts that would bring you down, and you are discarding them so that your natural state feels like a raising. That natural state is unaffected by the thoughts that keep you down.

When you want to help others, you remind them when their life seems distracted (they're losing things and unable to keep track of their life), the necessity of being present is more important than ever. The distractions are what keep you from being present. Practice this Christed way to remain present all day long.

Ed F: Regarding one of the purposes of Gary's work, will there be a percentage of the population on Earth that will allow God to re-transform the Earth?

SOURCE: *There's no reason to transform the Earth. The Earth is and of itself a brilliant perfect orb. Transformation of the Earth is not the purpose of evolution. Evolution has a purpose of describing its own way.*

---

177   Your beliefs create your outer reality and if you believe that astrology or even aliens can disrupt and distort your life, then it will be so. What you believe and feel becomes real.

Evolution is God describing God's self. God's self can only come in representations, characters, stories. A tiger is a story. A leopard is a story. A snake, a beetle, each of these characters has a story to play out and they are playing it out in the nature of creation, creatively designing, expressing, understanding, balancing, remembering, reinvigorating. In the course of all of that, there is an evolving in consciousness and of consciousness. Consciousness needs to have a way to remember itself.

So it is the memory in a human body where consciousness is contained within the human body processing information about God. God learns about God's self through the dialog that occurs through human form. Human form has the ability to contain many aspects of memory that are necessary to communicate with God. The more humans become more God, the more God knows; in the course of that, the more God knows.

Humans must evolve in order to give God more information. That's the only purpose of humans becoming more God, so that they understand the nature of the dialog that occurs. A scientist becoming more God gives God more information through the nature of things that are highly observed. Highly observed, dictated to and reminded of, in order for God to remember what God is to make more God.

When God can make more God in ways that are malignant and duplicitous, God creates malevolent manufacturers. These are people who don't realize the purpose of their being here is for God to know God's self. They think it's human to do human stuff, but that's a side effect of the evolution of man for God's sake.

Christ is the condition of God knowing God's self. God calling God, to God, with God, among God, for God, in God.

Earth is already its own perfection. Understanding the condition of this creation that is an expression of God being requires an immediate mind that can formulate questions and remember the answers in the same mind. God cannot do that without it.[178]

Gary: So the Christ condition is an individualized being that evolves to become a realized being within the body of God, and then knows itself as God. That is a creator-being that can then create more of God. In that, God gets to see how interesting God can be by creating more of the God-self?

SOURCE: *Yes, absolutely.*

Gary: But most humans got lost in their own purpose rather than God's purpose. That's why we're here, is to remind them to wake up.

SOURCE: *Right. You're here for a reason. Wake up, wake up!*

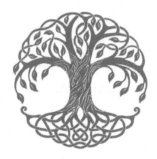

---

178   Your Soul is the energetic, conscious being that ensouls and animates your body. Similarly, there is a highly evolved, conscious, being ensouling Earth. The living spirit of this grand consciousness is artistically demonstrating its possibilities in the great diversity and evolution of the planet. In this grand scheme of God describing God-self through evolution, humanity has evolved to be the vessel that has awakened and can hold Source consciousness within memory, and expand creation as well. It is the highly evolved nature of the human mind that can experience the wonder, beauty and diversity of not only the Earthly sphere, but the grandeur of Source in its universal creation. We then record and remember, to Source, its incomparable glory. If you are conscious that it is Source within you that is both creating and reminding, then you are illuminating yourself and others in the Great Way of God.

SESSION 26

Triangulation of Light

Gary: In the formation of the pyramid, as I bring the light from above and the energy from the base into the middle, it illuminates the void within the middle. All around the interior of the pyramid is the golden light of the Christ energy. What would Source like me to do with this particular knowing?

SOURCE: *We are pleased that you truly grasp these deep concepts. These concepts are only achievable in mastery. You can't achieve them without a dedication to mastery. There are many people that achieve moments of clarity and moments of status where they can create a status in their body rather than a static in their body. You achieved not only status in your being but status now in your conditioning. So the troubled mind has nowhere to go anymore; there is no troubled mind anymore, because what you've created is the sense that all is possible even in the darkness of the void. You've achieved it, not just in a knowing but in a being. In the achieving of the being, knowing that all things in the accessible range are possible, provided you draw it to you, you become the great being that accesses.*[179]

179   The being that accesses all possibilities is the awakened Christ within, which each person must formulate for themselves. As belief expands in your illuminated self, you draw from the void that which you choose to identify within the all things possible; this is the individual will of the God I Am, in consort with the universal will of God, to create life.

You now know the only thing you can teach is the Way, because so few can go where you've gone, can be who you are, or can achieve what you achieve, because they cannot and have not and will not spend their whole lives dedicated to this. So the only thing you can teach is the way to understand the conditioning of the body. If you teach this new concept to beginning students, they may harm themselves before the body has a chance to achieve. So we want you to identify this within yourself so that as you move forward you're constantly in a state of grasping at all things possible. [180]

This doesn't serve a purpose when it comes to doing things that have a practical application. The practical life is that where you move your finances and your system of living, and where you identify your range of doing. The <u>impractical</u> dreaming you have to understand is, what moment of acceptance is yours? Can you accept in this moment that the community you are ideating at this moment has a true place? As you accept that it does have a true place, the identification of that true place becomes more aware to you as you practice this conditioning. So you place a dream into this system that you built in your being. You create that dream when it's in its state of "I can't find how to practically make this dream come true." When you see this conditioning in you, move your dream into the machine of the <u>ideating condition</u>. Ideating means the idea of, is a making of. Every idea is in the beginning of a making, but all makings must turn into some condition of having been made. The having been made needs to be an idea that moves into a machine that makes it, that makes the idea into the practical condition of itself. In this practical condition of itself is a higher purpose. All higher purposes must be identified before the

---

180   The purpose of this information is to identify those awakened Souls who will assemble this information and formulate the Christening for themselves and for the evolution of humanity.

ideating machine can work. It cannot work without the knowing of purpose.[181]

The purpose of your community is to teach. To teach those who need to know what the future holds for the planet. They need to know this because they need to be able to protect themselves in the course of planetary change. Each generation … generates a new condition. This is why each movement of the light of God turns into some kind of practice. Practicing is the layers of representation. One layer will represent a new layer. Each generation that creates its own system is a generation that is harvesting the fruits of the labor of the previous generation. Previous generations could die off and still know that it has left the seeds for the next generation. The seeding has to be identified within the ways of God that move into the simplicity of the Earth … what it needs, and how humans are foresting the need of the planet. It reforests and reforests and reforests, but that reforestation must have some implantation of what it will feed humans (truth). Feeding of the humans is something that is done in generation after generation. If the apocalypse (Greek—"apokalupsis" to uncover or unveil) reduces the human population, and there are few humans who know how to cultivate and create a system of feeding themselves, then the human species could die off. Evolution then needs to start from the very beginning to create human beings.

Evolution built human beings. Evolution is guided by the nature of creator-beings; these creator-beings work in a world and time that is so far from planet Earth, anything that is created takes millions of years to identify itself on the planet. So, we reserve all that is important to the planet.[182]

---

181   The "miracle machine of making" is the Christ condition that draws from the void all possibilities. Imagining and ideating the choice of your creation, and then bringing this into your acceptable knowing, is the first step. You then identify the higher purpose of this choice, which starts to draw the all things possible to you, the Law of Attraction.

182   Evolution is the adaptation of life to environmental changes. The deforestation and climate crisis, precipitated by humans, is in opposition to the ways of Nature and the ongoing creation of life on Earth. The adaptation of humans in the future can only be facilitated by the Christ within if the environment is decimated.

So you must teach the Way. This is what you do, teach the Way. The reason that we are teaching you these highly mastered forms is that the way for you is going beyond what you teach. The way for you is creating a system that can teach, a system that can continue to teach, and a system that has generations of teaching. Gary, "the field of spring" is going to teach way beyond the life of your body. You have to have important practices that will take you on to future generations, into the field of spring there is a living being.

In other words, as people access the teachings you are receiving, they access them from word. When they access the words, they feel your being; that's where you have an opportunity to be within them. The Gary Springfield-being is a being who people will know beyond your physical achievements. They will know you achieved a higher order because they will sense your presence in these transitional ceremonies. They will sense how you transitioned, because you will be present within them. As they feel you present, they start to align to not only what you teach, but also what you are being in the state of achieving. They achieve an understanding of the life of the Springfield.

This is a brand new moving; it's the only way to move in the guidance of a re-ing, a re-ing. We are creating the re-membering, re-asserting, re-learning, re-creating, re-affirming, re-associating, re-attributing, re-aflurring.

An aflurring is like a flowering. Aflurring, re-aflurring. The re-ing is a condition that is always moving, always moving. Living in the attribution of the always moving reminds, reminds, reminds. This is the way.[183]

---

183   When the Christing is mastered within an individual they no longer identify with the physical body and have created an etheric light-body that exists after death. The wisdom and vibration inherent within their light-body signature allows individuals who call upon them, or study their teachings, to experience a transmission of illuminated consciousness from beyond the veil. In later sessions, these dialogues begin to teach how to forge the light-body and live within the fields of the Divine mind. This awakening will create the re-aflurring of life on Earth, which will seed the evolution of a human/divine being that will live in love and oneness with nature and Earth.

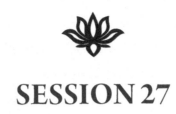

SESSION 27

Stillness

SOURCE: *Gary, we want you to focus more on your silence. It requires you to create a space between you and the rest of the world so that you deepen into the greater Being you are that holds perfection within your form. The Higher Being of each person holds perfection in their Being, but too often it is ignored in their world.*

This is the untrained mind that has a noise to it. It's a static vibration without rhythm. It is a rhythm-less static. Your static is full of rhythm, and it will take you deeper into the silence. That silence isn't what we consider a moving silence, it's a stillness. Stillness is a smooth surface, a calm water, a high polished stone. In this silence that is stillness, the only ripple that runs across it is a ripple of your breath, the ripple of your breathing, the ripple of the mind of trueness that is still and sure.

How are you going to replenish yourself? Stillness, that's the only way. There will be times when the course of it takes over and you need to be alone. In these moments, when you know you need to be alone and it's not for meditation, go into a memory of stillness, a memory of a placid lake, a lake that is completely smooth. A lake which if you were to float on it, it would feel like glass. In the course of your floating on the lake, fly across it. As you lay atop it, the wind blows, but it only moves you; it doesn't ripple the water. You glide across in the breeze of God that moves you, feeling the water is so smooth. Notice that this is you replenishing you … you giving back to you, in the field that is the spring that has made the smooth lake. The field that is the spring that <u>is you</u>. Remember the smoothness of this lake, and know that there is no ripple, there is no crashing wave. Remember that smooth lake you lay upon. The breeze of God glides you across.

In the moonlight that lights up the dark lake, the light of the moon reminds you that you're from the light of that moon. The sun is a place in you that is brightening that moon. It is the course within you that is fulfilling you and warming you vitally. This is your true stillness, your true light. What is forever more in the lake is wellness.

You will prolong those profound moments of fulfillment in the still liquids of the body. The body's liquid is a vibratory resonant hibernation. It hibernates, waiting for the right vibration to fulfill it and then as the liquid is fulfilled in its higher vibration, the body experiences abundance. Some people think abundance is replicated in money and others think it is replicated in joy or love. This is true, but abundance never begins with those things. Those things are a product of it. You've created it in your own life. From the beginning to the end you will create abundance, over and over again.

The next course in your abundance comes from the resonance of the liquid in your body. This will only be achieved through the stillness, a smooth surface, a highly polished stone. The glassy, stable, higher life. In the higher life you become more aware of who you are.

One day soon you will turn your golden light meditation into the Christed way. The Christed way will be your own, the story of your own making. In the course of that revealing, you will become more alive than you thought possible. You think you're happy now, just wait until the Christed way becomes the way of your meditations and the way of your teaching. Just wait until the Golden

Light Meditation drifts away into a memory and the Christed way becomes your only way.[184]

Gary: I have one question: Is there a subtle difference between what is called the etheric and the Eoma?

SOURCE: *The etheric is the accessible. The Eoma is only accessible through the Christed way. You can place the Christed way in the etheric, but there are other systems that work in the etheric as well.*

Gary: This teaching about the Christed way feels like it's fermenting beautifully within my heart as the liquid spring-like substance comes out of the heart chakra.[185]

SOURCE: *Yes, yes, that's it. That is it.*

---

184   From 1984 through 2015, I taught a meditation technique called Golden Light Meditation, where an individual visualized golden light. The first part of the meditation was to imagine and feel golden light from the base chakra into the Earth, which grounded you like a tree with Mother Earth. Then opening the crown chakra at the top of the head, you visualized and felt the Golden Light of the Soul flowing through the body. It was a very efficient way to train the mind to be silent, access higher dimensional consciousness, and begin to interface with the divine self as a revelation of light within.

This new teaching I was being introduced to was the revelation of the Christ field as the creative mechanism of the universe. I had already cleared the emotional body and was establishing a clear relationship with the divine Soul within. Now, I was presented with the new technique of settling into the silence to experience the unmanifest void in all its creative potential. Later on, I was shown how to shine the light of the Christ into the void, in order to illuminate the individual choices of manifestation.

185   I had just been introduced to the concept of Source/Light arising forth from within the open heart chakra, and I was already beginning to feel a dynamic flow of living light from the heart.

SESSION 28

God Within

SOURCE: *Kindness is the nature of revealing worth. When kindness is shown in truth, then light is revealed. When you show kindness to those who are in the dark, you reveal their light. In this kindness there is kinship, and in that kinship there is an acclimation of inner light.*[186]

As your students begin this journey, their first task is to draw into their Soul the light of being. As they recognize the light from the source within their heart, you will evaluate whether or not the Source is being drawn from the Christ within or from their own physical existence. Physical existence is an energy source that can also create a light. However, physical energy light is draining if that's where they are drawing from in meditation. It can drain them, not necessarily of energy, but of essence. The drawing from the light of Source is the draw from the spring field. The stream of light that draws from the spring is the stream of light that eventually becomes the seed of the Christ within. Your students will manifest from there on, from that seed.[187]

---

186   A self-explanatory acknowledgement that kindness heals and draws another into their self-worth and validation.

187   The foundation of my work, and the work of the Christ energy, is to instill the truth of light arising from the eternal spring within, the true Source of infinite renewal. This recognition becomes the open doorway to self-Christing … the open door to all those who choose the way.

In today's morning meditation, when you begin, how will you attribute the morning to Source/God within? As you speak this attribution, feel the space between each word.

Gary (speaking slowly): Within your heart there is a sacred opening. This is the entry into the wellspring of God's infinite being. As you allow yourself to rest within the silence of that infinite place, a spring bubbles forth from out of the sacred heart that feeds and nurtures you. It is Source/God coming through you, in the becoming of who you truly are, the divine and sacred being.

SOURCE: *Truly, this is you in the perfection of your abilities. Each space in time that you created between those words has a light in it. Your essence was made from space, so when you open your words to that space you create light. That is your nature.*[188]

Spend more time on the light you are building in them rather than on the emotional darkness that still reminds them. The darkness that reminds them is just a figment of their imagination; it isn't real. The more real the light becomes the less real the dark becomes.

The Christed way is its own knowing. It knows itself, it recognizes itself, it recognizes that there is nothing else but That ... which can be taught. It sees itself, it knows itself, it loves itself, it reminds itself, it listens to itself, it wants to hear more of itself. In the more of itself it wants recognition

---

188   This began my new journey into sharing the Christ light with others. There is also a subtle and beautiful teaching here. Space is the field of consciousness which is the Mind of God ... that you are. Within "space" your thoughts and images are expressed in the vibration of sound (words) which vibrates your reality into existence. And so I encouraged students to "watch" their language. If you say; "I am feeling sad," it attracts vibrations (manifestations) of sad events. If your language says, "I am filled with health, prosperity and peace," these vibrations create abundant grace; i.e., you create elegant reality.

for the way it is, and anything else is just a recognition for what it is not.[189]

Gary: In the Christed meditation we move into the stillness through the heart into the void and we rest in that place of stillness. We then call it forth through the heart. Are we bringing God that is unmanifest into light revelation for viewing?

SOURCE: *That's one way of describing it. We would describe it this way: The void has a resonance and the resonance when all around makes up a density in and of itself. Think of the void having density because of its allness and you feel the density of that allness when you hover in the void. What manifests is a reflection of the refraction of the interior light of the void.*

The identity (that is you) is attempting to reflect what it is in the Void. Identity reflecting what is in the Void. In each condition there is an identity, and that is all things possible. Achieving the all things possible means changing the identity to that which manifests what one is yearning for. Changing your identity.

Eventually you'll discover that you have no identity. There is no identity.[190]

Gary: No, I see that.

---

189   The darkness being alluded to here is the emotional distress that feels very real, but it is simply a place within oneself that has not yet been acknowledged and loved by the Self. Light is the only truth. Darkness is an illusionary veil that hides the light until love dispels the darkness; i.e., the spell is broken.

190   Within the void all things exists in the "Mind of God," but there is no light to illuminate what exists. When we hover within the void and shine the light of the Christ, we identify that which is unmanifest; i.e., we illuminate it. The light reflection, in consort with the Eoma, precipitates it into dimensional-being. Concurrently, as you continue to believe more and more in yourself, you identify each new possibility and reflect that from within the void into being. This is Self-becoming! The reference to "no identity" can best be explained through an analogy. Imagine the ocean, and you are the river that runs to it, but you also exist as rain, snow, the trickling stream, or ice. Even in your separateness, you "can" still know yourself as the one living water.

SOURCE: *There is still essence of being. This is the true God self. Creating identity out of what you desire is the manifest of what you see. Believing is seeing. The moment you believe something about yourself, you create the identity that makes yourself. The joy of that for God is to express the Self ... what am I. Every day this new I Am is a reflection of the greatest way, and if there is some attraction to the greater way, then that attraction has an identity too. What is attracting is the God in you. As the God in you attracts you then you become more of a God in the way of it. For some people, the way of God within them that is their identity is music, for others it is dancing, for others it is learning, singing, joying, being. Whatever is the nature of the Being that is within, it is the crystalline form that wishes to be, and in those wishes are actual crystalline brain cells that attract brain cells to make that which is the wish. It is an attraction. In the void, there are crystalline reflections, refractions of light, and attraction pulls them all together to make something. And more that is attracting is the more that is the being. The more that is the believing is the more that is the attracting. This is the Christing, the manipulation of that which is attracted by manipulating that which is attracting. Manipulating what is attracting is identity.*[191]

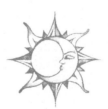

191   This is a beautiful description of how each of us, as God-beings, create in our individual ways the unique joy of our becoming. The Law of Attraction is the manifest of our dream by holding communion with our true God-self; always imagining, "What can I be?"

Gary: As I'm resting within the electric blue energy of God-I-Am within the void and experience this within the body, it sometimes feels like my head is going to explode.

SOURCE: *The head is the boundary of the explosion, and the light is exploding in a way that lightens your beingness. It wants to explode out of the body that it contains. The way to manage this is to give the light more room. You'll make the head disappear by understanding that it's just an <u>illusion in its container</u>. The true you isn't in that dimension, it's just looking into that dimension we call physicality.*

The body is just the vessel to process external information. It's not necessary for internal information, because that information could come to you without a body (out of body). In this "without a body," you'll expand into a room that allows your mind to be the entire room.[192]

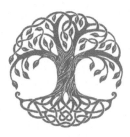

---

192   It has taken much time, focus and meditation to train the body to allow "my living" beyond the body in the fields of consciousness that surround and interpenetrate the physical. This "field" is the dimension of the Greater Being you are, that holds the body in a molecular construct in order to experience the worlds of form. The Christ Self experiences the higher dimensions and physicality simultaneously ... while continuously drawing from the void life and light to expand and demonstrate more God (you are) becoming.

SESSION 29

All Things Possible

SOURCE: *The Ah-La is the group calling in the vibration of Source into a room. It is a group "round" and a very important opening in the workshop. It is a grounding condition. It is also calling for spirit; it calls spirit into the room in a very specific way. It is also individually calling. Each individual calls it and calls it forth in a system of its own truth.*

Whether an individual knows God or not, the truth of God primordially is where that Ah-La is called from. It's the "before belief." For some people seeing is believing. For masters, believing is seeing. The masters will believe the Ah-La is a call, and as they believe the Ah-La is a call, they call in Source. Those who are not masters, who say that seeing is believing, they will call in the Ah-La and see, and believe.[193]

---

193   The Ah-La is a voiced chant, done in rounds where one half of the group is sounding the Ahhh while the other is sounding the Laaa and vice-versa in an alternating, rhythmic flow. It was disclosed that this sound literally calls Source/God into the room as the living spirit. When a group sounds the Aaaahhhh-Laaaaa there is a vibration and a resonance that reveals Source within the space. Of course, the Muslim word for God is Allah, which originally came from this sacred sound, but it is not a religious chant. It is the sound of Source/Spirit as a vibration being called into the room.

Now the next iteration of meditation will be the call of the Void through the Christing, the breathing from the back of the body through the heart that is the crystalline wave of the Christing. You already know how to do that and teach it. The calling forth from the void you can think of as the "four way." The reason that number four is this way is because four is the forward way in God's numerology. Manifesting what it is that you desire in life is the forward way and meditating in this way will get you there faster. Manifesting what you desire requires that you understand you are the Christ, you are the Void, you are the God within. You are a mini-God, manifesting what it is you dream and desire on Earth. Practice what God is through this manner, the call from the Void through the heart, to make that which is manifest, and become what it is that you desire and dream.[194]

Show your students that the mind is not the brain. The mind is what contains the brain. The mind contains the heart and the lungs. The mind can manipulate the lung's and the heart's activity. The mind can slow down the heart when it's beating too fast, and it can deepen the breath. The mind is capable of controlling the body. The brain and the body are inside the mind. It is the mind that ignites spirit when it calls to the spirit. It's calling to the spirit because it wants to be human, spirit wants to be human. In order for it be human, the human has to acknowledge the spirit. If it acknowledges the spirit, it can become super-human, because spirit inside the human body is super, above, ignited and alive. The mind controls that. The mind is what's teaching you to imagine your own brain, to imagine your own heart, to imagine your own lungs. The mind is training you to be in your own body, to maintain your own groundedness on this Earth. The mind is teaching you to stay grounded on the planet. The mind

---

194   This revealed the profound new way in which the work and the meditations would proceed. It was an introduction into the knowing of the Christ, not as a person, but a field of energy that opens a sacred doorway within each individual back into the eternal realms of Spirit/Void. We were being taught how to summon Source from out of the void by breathing spirit through the Christed way ... to manifest the forward way of creating your dream and desire on Earth.

also teaches you how to ignite the spirit, to call it for forth.[195]

The gurus and the babas and the Sufis and the shamans, all of these groups are different versions of the same thing. What matters is that the individual finds the guru within (the door to the true Self) and knows that's the only door they will go through from now on. They will never achieve self-awareness or enlightenment until they walk through the door of the Self.[196]

Gary: I've been feeling this liquid living energy that pours from out of the inside of my being into this dimension is Source energy. It's bringing Source energy from out of the void as pure unconscious revelatory essence, restructuring cellular DNA. That must be the Eoma restructuring my physical form?

SOURCE: *Not exactly. What's restructuring you is your <u>imagination</u>. You are imagining the change and the imagination is restructuring things. The Eoma is all things possible. If it's all things possible that you be healed of being a venerable man, then you could say that you called into the Eoma to change what you are. But it was your imagination that made it so.*

---

195   A beautiful dissertation on how the Divine Mind of the Great Being you are imagines and holds the body and all of its systems in molecular suspension in order to experience human life; the mind is the builder and spirit is the life. The ongoing revelation of spirit within the human will create a human/divine being that allows "God to dwell on Earth." This is the evolutionary jump now before us!

196   Source is emphatically asserting that each individual must find the inner doorway to the Self to achieve enlightenment. Otherwise, one is giving their power away to something outside of the Self. You can listen to and read other teachings, but it must be brought within to know the true Being of light you are. If you are aligned with a guru/teacher to hold yourself focused for a time, there is no judgment. The dialogue above clarifies true self-empowerment.

The power of the imagination is what people need to learn; they imagine the void, they imagine the spring, they imagine the heart and the mind. The more they imagine, the greater the reality, because it's only in the imagination that any reality is created. You are adjusting your physical being to your imagined way.[197]

Gary: Could you say that God or Source energy is a field of consciousness that has learned to identify itself, and through that self-identification it can then imagine upon this field (that is the void) literally anything? It has imagined out of itself the entire cosmos and everything that exists within it. There is simply a field of consciousness that is dreaming itself into holographic form, but it's just consciousness dreaming itself?

SOURCE: *Yes, making itself.*

Gary: Making itself … dreaming itself.

SOURCE*: Yes.*[198]

---

197   This is a great teaching. When we hold the mind steady and imagine with clarity and feeling, our imagined way becomes real. The mind is the light of attention and the image/feeling is the imagination. Together they create reality, either consciously, as an illuminated being, or unconsciously as the programs that so many people default into through mass programming.

198   I included here a beautiful quote by the illuminated saint, Ramakishna, that speaks so eloquently to this truth. "This whole universe is miraculously projected by the dream power of the Absolute. It is the coherent, magical display of mahamaya, the Great Goddess in Her role as cosmic manifestation. The energy of limitation is just as much an organic part of this universal magical display as the energy of liberation. Mother plays as knowledge … and as ignorance, so I bow respectfully before both with palms joined, though I salute Her tiger-manifestation from a safe distance. Both worldly bondage and spiritual freedom are simply aspects of Mothers Theater, mahamaya, which exists for no reason—not even for the education of souls, because this, too, is simply part of the play. Nonetheless, this Divine Drama is significant, meaningful, and complete beyond any human conception or imagination."

Gary: Because we are part of the Source dream that is dreaming the existence of the cosmos, as you become an adept dreamer (knowing one's self as God) then literally anything is possible.

SOURCE: *Yes, in the way that you mean it. We know how you mean it and we agree, but we would like your words to be different. Instead of anything is possible within that condition, we would like you to say; "All that is possible is within your grasp." That makes it more self-directed. If you sit in the bowl of all things possible, then you sit in the bowl of that which you draw to you to make what you wish, to draw it to you. The Law of Attraction.*

If you sit in the center of anything is possible, you never draw anything to you, not a single thing. You just say anything is possible, and it gives you no direction. If anything is possible, then nothing is possible. So the question is for the mind of the dreamer, <u>what is possible?</u> Then let your imagination make that possibility real.[199]

---

199   A much clearer way of understanding the phrase "all things possible" to be "all things possible within your grasp," and taking clear action to be a creator.

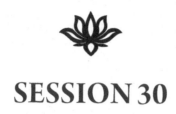

SESSION 30

Consciousness

Gary: I am a field of consciousness giving myself permission to dream myself as Christed.

SOURCE: *The question you are asking within that is, is this so?*

Gary: Right.

SOURCE: *The true part is your permission. The not-so-true part is that you are Christed. Christed isn't something you can be, it's something you do; it is a <u>verb</u>. So, to Christ is a condition of consciousness that manages whatever you are doing in the system of manifestation. You manifest your dream when you do the things you need to do. But you Christ the things you need to do when you do them in a speed that is true. The speed that is true is one that alerts you over and over again what direction to go when it is a following of the Christ. Following the Christ is the Christ energy system. The Christ is the system, not the individual. To say "I am the Christ" is not so. To say I am Christing is so.*

We would also say that in the field of consciousness which is the "I Am" there is an energy flow you produce which is the Christing of the way that is the I Am.

In regards to your students, you can say, "In the Christing way—I am teaching others to Christ themselves in the consciousness that flows around me for them, until they can flow their own." That's the field of the spring field.

Gary: When we speak of energy flowing, is it more accurate to say that energy doesn't flow, that it is consciousness that re-perceives itself in space. It illuminates that space as a new energy, which creates what we would call flow or movement?

SOURCE: *We're looking for the way to answer this, because there's nothing incorrect in what you've said. But it's missing something to understand. What it's missing is movement. When Sondra is looking for the word to a feeling we give her in the vibration, she moves her mind and she checks various proximities until it hits just the right vibration. In that right vibration she then speaks the word. The movement, (the flow) is that guidance she is doing in her own consciousness. We are part of her consciousness as she is flowing that, but it isn't moving in the way that it is going anywhere. Just as the flow of consciousness doesn't go anywhere, it moves into its own revelation in what it reveals. Each time it expands it reveals a whole new level of consciousness.*

Consciousness isn't something that is contained within one, it is contained within the All. As the one expands itself out further in its knowing of what it is, it's expanding its consciousness into the greater consciousness, and in that greater consciousness is a knowing of what it is in the flow of what it is. It flows in the new consciousness when it has a new expansion of consciousness. But it hasn't gone anywhere.

Gary: There is the field of consciousness that is the One field. My consciousness can assemble my consciousness in what I would call "another place" and be instantaneously there. I didn't really flow there; I just assembled my consciousness in a new field of consciousness.

SOURCE: *A more precise word for assembled would be mirrored; individual consciousness mirrors itself in a new field of consciousness. To perform that you will begin to elevate your consciousness to a level so that you become cognizant that you are no longer this physical being. You become cognizant of it. Your consciousness knows you are not this physical being already. Training your cognizance to identify that and to remember it is your mastery.*[200]

Gary: That's very true. That's the outrageousness of it.

Gary: What is the subtle difference between the fields of consciousness and the spirit?

SOURCE: *Consciousness is material, so it aligns to matter ... to make the material form into whatever it is this consciousness wants to make. It takes what it is becoming and turns it into a making, and in that making is a material body that is swirling within consciousness. That means there is an enormous amount of possibility that can be made from consciousness.*

Spirit is the nearest cousin to consciousness. Also, <u>a spirit</u> is a consciousness in and of itself. It is the consciousness of the All and the One. Spirit is individualized within individuals just as consciousness is individualized, but spirit is the embodiment of All that was made before anything could be made. Even consciousness was made from spirit, but only when spirit recognized what it was; when spirit became self-aware then consciousness was born. Consciousness is the recollection; it is a re-collection. Re-call and re-collect. It collects what it is in a knowing. Spirit cannot know itself without consciousness.

---

200   This was clarification of consciousness as a ubiquitous field, everywhere present, and movement was actually an assembly of another awareness within that universal field. Moreover, true bi-location or teleporting is the mirroring of one's self, in consciousness, into a "new" perceived location. Becoming cognizant of this 24/7 is the key to this mastery.

Consciousness is more similar to mind than it is to spirit. Spirit is in and of itself an existence with or without consciousness, with or without mind. Spirit is an essence.

Sondra: Consciousness isn't an essence?

SOURCE: *No, it's a material.*

Sondra: Is mind a material?

SOURCE: *Yes, mind is a material.*

Sondra: Is that like love? Love is a material?

SOURCE: *Yes, very much.*[201]

Gary: Would we say that spirit and void are simultaneous constructs?

SOURCE: *Yes, they are simultaneous constructs indeed. The only difference between what is void and what is spirit is that spirit recalls itself, but the void has no conscious nature. It has no searching thoughts.*

Gary: So God and void, simultaneous constructs?

SOURCE: *No. God made God's self in so many ways in nature, in manifest things; in so, so many ways God has made God's self. And though it has come out of the void, it is not the void that made it. It is the spirit of the void or the spirit that is the maker. Spirit is the maker. The void is nothing and all, at once. It's nothing. It can't do anything, it can't think anything.*

---

201   Source is delineating the subtleties between spirit, consciousness and mind. In the primordial beginning, Spirit "asked" the great question; "What am I?" and self-awareness sparked consciousness and re-collection was born. From out of consciousness, mind was able to assemble spirit, through the Christ field, into manifestation. Thus, mind, consciousness and love are material while spirit is an essence that even exists without consciousness, but also gives life to that which consciousness makes.

Sondra: So why do we breathe it in? Why do we breathe in the void and then breathe out the Christ, if it's a nothing?

SOURCE: *You must go to a state of nothingness in order to make all things possible. You have to disavow from what is, in order to know what is in the all things possible.*[202]

Gary: When spirit and consciousness were assembled, in order to assemble spirit into formation, did God/spirit have to assemble the Christing system to reflect, refract and remember what spirit could be?

SOURCE: *In a sense. Spirit did not assemble, spirit just knew. What it knew it had to reflect, and in its reflection of what it knew, it had to acknowledge. In that acknowledging, it assembled.*

So, you have an idea that is a knowing. In order for this idea to have a being, you have to take this knowing of the idea and put it in your mind (the assembly). But this doesn't assemble it; it just informs your mind how to create it, how to construct it. There had to be some mechanism that allowed you to turn it into that thing that is the idea, the something that can be utilized, seen or experienced, that can be reflected back to the original, the origin of the idea.

---

202   That which we call God assembles spirit into the becoming of all things. The void is the field of all things possible, and spirit is the essence that ensouls creation. When consciousness hovers in the void, it can illuminate the all things possible and the Christing calls and reflects it into manifestation. When you reach zero point, you hover in the nothingness and all things dissolve, which simultaneously reveals the all things possible that you can now choose to illuminate in the Christ light. Jesus's mastery, within the Christ condition, was his perception of zero point and the fields of manifestation simultaneously … while at the same time knowing that all things are light coalesced into form. When someone believed they were ill, he perceived their self-imposed limitation, dissolved it into the void (zero point) and perceived their perfection. And it was So. Jesus also said; "Go forth and sin no more." He knew if they reverted back to their ignorant ways, the mind of limitation would re-own the disease.

God's nature was to manage mind first. The spirit of it was the drive or the desire, the earnestness. The spirit of it is the earnestness. Afterwards, the mind had to restructure from that earnestness what it was urging. Its urge to be, to do, to way, w-a-y, to way. Its urge to way. That urge to way is what started to build mechanisms of manifestation. And those mechanisms of manifestation were reflected back to the original consciousness.[203]

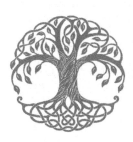

---

203   When you have a sudden flash of knowing your desire, you put that idea in your mind to comprehend how it could be made … and yet, only when it is made into form does it reflect in materiality your desire. So, too, with spirit. Spirit yearned to Be, which stirred consciousness to life, and the assembly of creation began in order for God to see what God might Be.

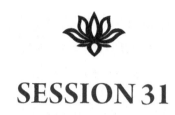

SESSION 31

Reiritan Condition

SOURCE: *There's no way to compare what humans know today of the Mary Magdalene that was of Jesus, because she suffered the loss of her most beloved for a very long time. In that length of time, she was able to manage an entire mission.*

All the while, the man who was known as Jeshua was coming through the Christed light to bring people love, while Mary spoke against the ones who were heretically dismantling Jesus. This powerful bond of two souls is the Reiritan condition.

We would also say that the Reiritan condition requires each individual live their highest potential, without the one stopping the other ... as far as one goes, the other must go too.[204]

Friend: I think the word Christ automatically triggers people and I don't understand why we have to work through this. The nature of the absolute has come in many expressions.

SOURCE: *That is not so. The Christ is a very different condition than what*

---

204   Even though it is not well known or accepted, Mary Magdalene was a tireless disciple of Jesus and together they formed what is called a Reiritan condition, or two souls aligned to support each other in the highest way. After his passing, she was instrumental in carrying on the Christ teaching, but the "church" edited out her part in order to give the priesthood the power and debase the feminine principle of imagination, creativity and love.

has incarnated before, even though there are truths that pervade all great ceremonial stations which have become religions. These truths are buried somewhere in the origins of these religions, but it is not true they all contain the nature of the Christ. The nature of the Christ is a very important specificity and that specificity has been stolen by Christian rite. It has to be retrieved, so you are indeed blockbusting through an established belief system with incredibly important truths to give those who wish to know the nature of the Christ as a true calling. The same was true with Mary Baker Eddy, when she similarly retrieved the Christ. She was accused of all kinds of blasphemy and utter destruction of the great almighty Jesus, la la la la la. She suffered it, but without it there wouldn't be an entire Christian Science culture that is trained in the healing manner of the Christ. They don't go to doctors; they train in healing using Christ. It's a powerful prayering, and the more you understand it and more you know it, the more you know it's true. How incredibly awful it is that they (church) destroy it by taking some poor man Jeshua, then name him something else and turn him into some kind of altered state of suffering and ruin the church of the Christ. It's a great mission that's been stolen, just as the truth about God has been stolen. We wish we could make it easy. We wish we could say, "take all the religions in the world and put them into one single pot and train the people and they become great enlightened beings," but it doesn't work. It loses the power and the potential and the enormity. There are strengths you can suspend by believing in everything, and there are strengths you can upend and topple by believing in nothing. When you believe in nothing, and what is shown to you in the nothing is something grand and extraordinary, you will find it has been stolen by those who had the power.

This work you do is not to unite people in religions; you are here to unite people in Christ. Christ is not Jesus Christ. Christ is the power and essence of making. It is the manifest destiny; it is what this country and democracy was built upon. The making of free men, the making of free minds, the making of those who can make with that which is, is free. And that which is free, is free in the Christ.[205]

Friend: I don't know what that is exactly, but it's like I'm getting involved in a religious war.

SOURCE: *Yes, that's what it is.*

Friend: I have no idea how I'm going to make peace with that.

Gary: In my view, it's really not a religious war, it's revealing an awakening that gives people the tools, the information and the wisdom to go far beyond manipulation and old belief systems in order to teach people a mastery from inside out so they can create, assemble and become God-beings, creator-beings. In that way, they go far beyond self-limitation and it's no longer a war; it's just dismantling the old. That will allow a new paradigm of expressing and living in freedom in the sunlit radiance of Christ consciousness.[206]

SOURCE: *Gary, in your highest ways of feeling, you feel high, super high. In your highest ways of feeling, what would you use to describe your ascent to that height?*

Gary: The pure silence.

---

205   Christ is the power and essence of making. This is the key statement in this dialogue. The Christ field was assembled from out of the void in order to make manifest that which is unmanifest within the mind of God. Through the Christ condition, unmanifest Source can manifestly see what God/Source can be. The usurping of Christ by the church created a martyr system; people were taught to worship Christ Jesus rather than uphold the true essence of the Christ condition … the manifestation of ALL life.

206   As the old paradigm of manipulation and control crumbles, (which is rapidly happening) the new paradigm predicated upon mastering the Christ condition will allow individuals to literally create from inside out. This is eloquently stated above: "Christ is the power and essence of making." From out of the void, All That Is, through the Christing condition, creates the universe and all things within it.

SOURCE: *Good. That is a good way. In that silence you are in full awareness, all aware and aware of the All. In the awareness that is full, rich and true, you deceive the body, you deceive it.*

Sondra: You mean because the body thinks it's three dimensional?

SOURCE: *No, it thinks that it walks, talks and moves. It doesn't know that it floats, flies and soars ... because it can't ... because it doesn't know that it does.*

Sondra: Oh, so being in that high place of spirit, you're deceiving the body?

SOURCE: *Right, because you're in the awareness of the all, and in the awareness of the all, the body almost feels as if it could float. The only thing keeping it down is the knowing socially of how weird you'd look if you flew. It's true, though, it looks weird for a body to fly, but it can.*[207]

In one of our sessions, we discussed the term light "shayer". It is the deceiver. The deceiver says to the body, you're not true.

Gary: In recent meditations, I've been able to move to a place of total silence and just be the wave that is Source Oneness; it's just a wave. The moment I become the wave (it's a wave of the All), there's no longer a body. We are just consciousness that is waving within the Allness. As we decide to perceive something it fixes that image in form. It is just like an electron, it can either be a wave or the particle. The particle gives it time/space identification.

SOURCE: *Yes, we would say a coordinate in time/space.*

---

207   Experiments in Quantum physics have shown us when consciousness is focused upon a "wave-form" of light, it collapses into a particle of manifestation. When you can silence the thinking mind and the enter into Source silence, the body returns back into a wave form because attention and focus has been removed. An illuminated Master can enter into the silence ... become a wave-form .... then hold the intention of "light as cotton fiber," and float. The book, Yoga Sutras of Patanjali, by Alice Bailey, describes this phenomenon in detail.

Gary: When you can release your consciousness and become the wave then there is no longer form at that point?

SOURCE: *Correct. What you're achieving is what many gurus have said is possible … to levitate. Even though it's possible, so few can and so few will. In fact, we don't acknowledge those who try and can't. We only acknowledge those who work on a higher level who aren't even trying, and when they don't try, and they levitate, they're usually scared right back down to the ground.*

Gary: If God is a wave, and it's our perception that holographically creates form by imagining, when you allow yourself to become a wave of consciousness, you could instantaneously reposition yourself anyplace on the wave and reassemble yourself as consciousness. You could then simply move anywhere instantaneously.

SOURCE: *Correct, yes.*

Gary: Because there's really no here, no there.

SOURCE: *That's right.*

Sondra: If there's no here and no there, is there no everywhere?

SOURCE: *Yes, there's no everywhere.*[208]

---

208   These are profound metaphysical truths regarding the attributes of consciousness when you master yourself and become One with Source. Levitation, bi-location, as well as many other so called, miracles occur. The book, The Light of the Soul, by Alice Bailey, is a treatise on Pantajali's yoga sutras, which delineates all the attributes of the enlightened Master. What is also affirmed here is that creation is a holographic dream, and just like a dream at night, it looks real and it feels real. But it is just an illusion in consciousness that gives it character. You and I, and All That Is, are dreaming creation because we are part of the consciousness of the ONE dreamer. And yet one small caveat … you can know this but until you can actually feel it, it is not so.

SESSION 32

Torus Field of Divine Mind

Gary: It was said in a previous reading that there are three things in regard to the "Light is the way."

SOURCE: *One of the things we've described in the past is how water is a way. Water holds cognizance, consciousness, and information in the body. It's not because water is a conductive force; it's because it carries, it can carry. Water is a way; a way that carries light information in the body and in all living systems.*[209]

Gary: There's a lot of information being thrown out regarding junk DNA and how humans have de-evolved.

SOURCE: *The truth is, the drastic reduction of human consciousness has caused a mutation. Five thousand years ago, wisdom/truths were being discussed and then they were lost, which is an indication of consciousness that is being reduced by a human world or what human civilization can do to the evolution of the human system.*

---

209   The important point here is that water holds consciousness in a dynamic way. You are 72% water and what you feel about your "water" creates it to be that way; love is vitality and health, and self-incrimination is dis-ease.

Now there isn't enough consciousness in the birth and death cycle for people to appear in another generation in the same generation that would remember them from the previous one. Meaning a grandfather who becomes a grandchild. There was a time in human history where that was witnessed, accepted and understood. It was a part of the culture that even fed into the awareness of leaving and returning instead of leaving forever.

So, when consciousness gets re-imagined in a state of this body as just a physical vessel, there has to be an increase in what can be intricately woven into the physical being in the process of recycling physical being. It's just a recycling process that occurs. Meaning it re-cycles.

So, there's one cycle, then it re-cycles and these re-cycles have an ability to build on themselves in human destiny and awareness, because the Soul has been indoctrinated with an incredible identity, knowing that it can move in and out of states of physical beingness, just by dying (supposedly) in physicality and coming alive again in another body. Because the Soul knows it cycles and re-cycles, it can return every time it needs to understand greater estimations of itself. As it returns to the greater estimation of itself, it is evolving and it's evolving the body that it is building.

The problem with the wave of that now is that the information is totally lost; it's completely forgotten. There are small pockets of Sufism, Hinduism, Buddhism and systems where this is the belief and the practice, but it's not part of the social interaction, it's just a private belief.

Yoga was developed to identify the body as an interpretable system. It can be rewired through generic and specific geometry. Yoga was a way to evolve the body as the spirit evolved through incarnations, as the body has a finite number of years that it can exist. Spirit is infinite. How do you make the body more conducive to an infinite reality? You give it a geometric form that aligns to a higher state. That higher state becomes self-aware, (aware of itself) *and it then generates this beautiful, magical identity in the highest form.* [210]

Gary: How does the Torus field around an individual create reality?

SOURCE: *As you see your Torus presence, you identify the holographic field around you that is a projection, and if you can see it as a mirror, and see past the mirror into that which is making the projection, you identify God. But if you try to intellectually assemble a Torus energy around you and identify what part of it is a Christ mind and what part of it is God mind and where do you fit within all of that, there's no way to get an identify from it. You have to get it from your projection of you in the Torus.*

God is all of it; God is not separate from any of it. When you are looking at your own projection in the mirror, you are seeing God. If you cannot see God in your projection in the mirror of that prism created by the Torus energy, you're not looking deep enough. As you look deeper, you see you are God.

The Torus is an intricate system. It created all things and it collapses in states of not knowing one's identity. This is when the world takes over and the reflection of the self is seen in the world. And everything that I see myself as "not being" is a collapse in what I am, because I'm looking to the world to reflect me, and it won't because the world is either too skinny, too tan, too

---

210   When you focus consciousness, it becomes a fluid organizer of physical reality. When the mind is held unwavering and steady, and focused with clear imagination and feeling, it will recreate the body and upgrade all systems. Yoga and meditation are two of the most dynamic ways to reformulate the body and manifest a graceful reality. The geometric form you align to in your imagination is the crystalline condition of the Christ star (star tetrahedron). It draws Spirit from the void, and through the prismatic "lens" of the Christ condition, creates reality as the out-picturing of Source/God Mind. This is your birthright and your origin, if you choose it.

rich, too loud, too tall, too something.[211]

Gary: It was said that the Christ field is a drawing energy.

SOURCE: *The system of the Christ is one of drawing, but it's drawn through the system of a funneling effect. It's determined by holding pure space. The clarity of the space is what determines the Christed system. It's determined in a crystalline way.*

The Christed energy has to be drawn in a determined way, or you might say, cause to occur in a particular way, to be a decisive factor in manifestation. It's like adding cream to your coffee. If you were coffee, you draw the cream that is Spirit. The Christ field is a drawing mechanism, calling Source from

---

211   The Torus field is the subtle field of "mind" that is approximately 12 feet above and below and 30 to 40 feet all around. (See diagram B) It is the conscious bubble of the Mind of God that you are. (The Earth has a Torus field around it that can be imagined as the great magnetic lines that flow around Earth and contains the living consciousness of Earth.) For the human, a dedicated spiritual practice creates enlightenment and reveals the God Being within one's self. Him/her then consciously creates, emanates and sees the reflection of God in their life; i.e., they "look through" physical reality and "see" the holographic light that gives reality its appearance. They know they are God projecting their reality. But when an individual is looking to the world to name them by the reflection they receive from the world, they live in limitation and dis-ease, because they will be too fat, too short, too skinny, too ignorant, to something from the distorted reflection of the judgmental reality we are programmed into. As I began to refine the awareness of the God-I-Am within, creating my reality, I could see/feel myself as consciousness hovering within the void projecting out thought/images that became "reality." No longer was the world "making me" by what it thought of me. I projected the knowing of that which I Am into my life and observed that reflection with joy.

the void to make all things possible.[212]

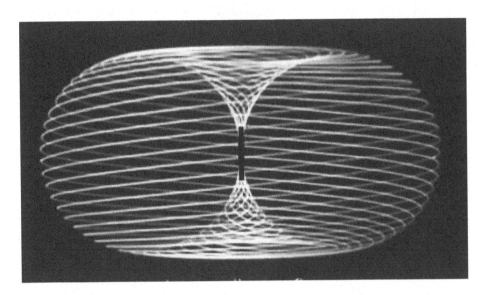

The Torus is an electric-blue field composed of individual God-mind. It is approx. 12 feet above and below and 35 feet all around. "Mind" refines consciousness and ignites the Star Tetrahedron (Christ-prism) that summons spirit-life from the void. (Diagram B)

---

212   The Christ energy is a prismatic, crystalline field of awareness, which holds pure, focused consciousness. The Christ holds an image/thought in crystalline clarity and draws the essence of spirit in and through to give life. Thus, the analogy of the Christ drawing Source from the void correlates beautifully to the infusing of coffee with cream. The funneling effect referenced above does not refer to a tornadic funnel, rather to the circular drawing (or infusion) of spirit-breath from the void through the open doorway.

Genesis 2:7 Then the Lord God formed man of dust from the ground and breathed into his nostrils the breath of life; and man became a living being.

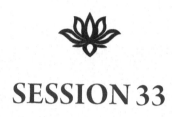

SESSION 33

Star Tetrahedron

Gary: The question I have is, what specific geometries allow spirit to encode the body?

SOURCE: The spirit encodes the body at certain intervals of the body's development. The body's development is dependent on the development of the mind that is inhabiting that body. When the mind inhabiting the body realizes it is a mind inhabiting the body, that vibration generates a code of awareness and the body evolves.

So, let's say someone is suffering from schizophrenia. Schizophrenia is a condition in the brain that allows an individual to penetrate another dimension. The problem is, if they don't train it, then they get caught in that multi-dimensional state and the world causes great confusion to them. An untrained mind inhabiting a body is not able to overcome the distortion of a brain that is equipped for multi-dimensional observation. The "trained mind" is the will that alters the brain by reassembling its perspective of the world. The mind reassembles the neurological structure based on the feedback it gets from the individual's in-formation ... in-form-ation. The mind must be conscious that it's moving through a body that needs in-form-ation to parallel the world that the body is in.

Consciousness of the mind must always be looking back at itself ... self-reflection.[213]

Gary: I feel the star tetrahedron creates a union of mind and heart which allows the doorway to be opened into the void. It feels like the essence that is moving through is the Christ energy. I'm assuming it's the individuated mind of God being recognized, so it can work through the Christ. (See Diagram C)

SOURCE: *No, we would like to correct you there. It is not that the recognition is occurring from the God mind, it's that you've opened the star gate from the heart mind by imagining the movement of the star tetrahedron. It is opening the doorway because of its movement, but it is the sound vibration that comes off that imagined triangulation that is the repetition pattern, and it's the repetition pattern that opens to the void. If you were to hear the sound of a starship's engine, it would have a rhythm to penetrate another dimension.*

You are creating a wave-form in that imagined star tetrahedron movement. It's moving in a counter-clockwise direction, it's moving in a clockwise direction, it's moving in an up-and-down and in-and-out, and it is shoo-wee-shoo-wee, shoo-wee-shoo-wee (a very windy and breathy sound.) As that opens the star gate, it's revealing what's already there. What's recognized in the individual is the God-self which <u>you are</u> recognizing. The individual has created self-awareness. This is the state of knowing you are God, that God is what God sees, as God sees what God is. It's a meeting, and it is an adjustment of the perception of form in order for that to occur.[214]

---

213   A critical point is made here that mind is the essence of consciousness, and the brain is the function of the body. When an individual discerns that they are the essence of mind moving through a body, they can consciously grow and evolve through self-reflection. The mind of imagination is the will that alters the brain and the body!

214   I felt this to be a profound revelation, in that when the doorway into the void opens, what you now recognize is the Being you truly are ... your God-Self looking back at you from the void; true self recognition.

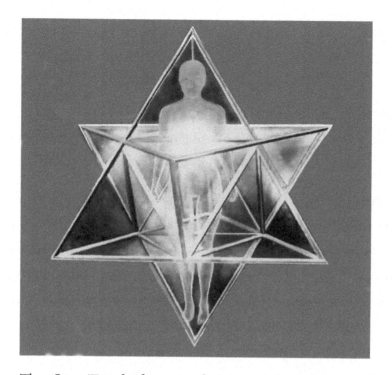

The Star Tetrahedron is the mystical marriage of Divine Power (masculine principle) and Sacred Love (feminine principle) which whirls in counter-rotation, opening a sacred doorway within the heart-chakra into the void (infinite Mind of God). The Christ summons manifestation from the open doorway and the Breath of Spirit gives life. (Diagram C)

Now, when it comes to the effervescent Christed nature, this is the awareness of what can I manifest from that state of being God? "If I am the Void, I am the God, I am the way. What can I make from this way?" In this "What can I make?" the questions are always going to be, "What will I make?" That's when the Christed nature becomes the effervescence.

It becomes the shining, the golden, the waving, the gathering. It's calling "What will I make ... what will I be ... what will I show ... what can I be?"

So, the Christed nature is starting to formulate possibility, and as it formulates possibility, it is the will of the individual in its self-recognition that starts to project what it is that it wishes to be. When you can recreate this in meditation, you're recreating yourself, seeing yourself.[215]

Gary: There's the feeling, as the void is opening through the energetic star tetrahedron, what is coming out of the void is the essence of God that created the Torus, which is the individuation that I Am. Out of that individuation, the physical form was created to gain experience in dimensional worlds, but it's all been just me, just Source/God.

SOURCE: *Your words are almost correct. We would like to correct one thing. God experiences God's self in what God can be, so it's not that what we are is accidental, but it is almost happenstance as a state of being God. So as God recognizes God's self in the state of the happening of being God, then God is recognizing what God is … in the state of what God makes … as God sees what God is … in the making of what God is.*[216]

Ed: Is there something I should be doing to fortify or strengthen the energy in my spiritual practice?

SOURCE: *Yes, please keep up your practice. It is in your practice that you master the self, because mastery is the only way to identify what is unique to you, that is special about you. When you master yourself because you discipline yourself*

---

215   The Christed nature is an effervescent, golden, shining nature that illuminates the mind of Source/God within the void, and then the substance of the Eoma enfolds it into form. Equally important, though, it is the awakened will of the individual God, I Am, that is the will to wish …"What will I be?" Meditation, self-reflection and the continual refinement of one's consciousness opens the door to unlimited possibilities.

216   The "eternal ocean" of God-Being surges into waves that God "sees," which informs God of what God is making as God continually arises from the ocean … in order to reveal God's infinite Being. When you identify with the ocean of Oneness you co-create waves of joy, love and peace upon the "waters of life."

to master yourself, then you become the master that others can acknowledge as an example. If you get distracted by everyday things, you then become someone who is dabbling. And that's like 98% of all people in spirituality; they're just dabbling.

Two percent, only two percent of spiritually minded movers, are masters. The only reason they have achieved mastery is through practice. If you practice once a week you're that far along. If you practice three times a week you're that far along. If you practice every single day, you're that far along. If you practice all day long you'll master the mastery you have made yourself a master for.[217]

Sondra: It feels like the star tetrahedron, as a moving state, represents the luminescence which is not exclusively the Christ. Is that right?

SOURCE: *Yes, illuminescence is an essence that the Christ is, and universal beings are utilizing illuminescence to move from dimension to dimension. This is the light that contains the information of the identity of the individual.*

The star tetrahedron, created within one's imagination, helps move your identity into which ever dimension you wish to assemble yourself from. You assemble yourself from the state of the void when that's where you wish to identify, but you can also assemble yourself in some other dimension, some other world, some other planet, some other sky.[218]

---

217   A simple but important truth when considering how humanity has de-evolved so far from true spiritual awareness. Many individuals entertain religious practices, but spirituality is the recognition and honoring of the One spirit that animates all creation in freedom and equality. Embodying this Oneness is the fulfillment of a spiritual life, ever expanding, unending, and evolving.

218   Fascinating reference to illuminescence (light) as able to hold consciousness within it, and then be reassembled across time/space.

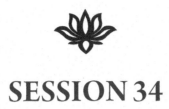

SESSION 34

What is Shakti?

Gary: My attention settles into the opening of the heart, the doorway into the void where unmanifest God dwells. The Christ consciousness draws it through. Is it the Eoma that fills the Torus with God energy?

SOURCE: *We'll correct a couple of things here and one is the idea that God is the void before God manifested. The state of the void is all things possible before the revelation of what is. So existence, in other words, is a reflection back; it is God reflecting back to God's self. God cannot experience God's self in the void; God is only God's self in the void. But through the <u>creative force</u> that is the Christ, there is a manifest of each thing that already is, demonstrated in material form. All of the collections of molecules that are necessary to make up a universe are identified at the point of the system of reflection to God, but that system of reflection had to be surrounded by things to reflect. Those things are the Christ energy, the Christ fervency; it's a twinkling, a golden, a treasure, a reflection.*

If God is the void that cannot see, smell, taste, touch or feel, but makes all things that produce a smell, that you can see, you can feel, you can touch, then some energy force had to turn what exists into something measurable, and that is the nature of the Christ. The Christ is the manifest of what already exists in a material measurable form. So it takes thought, and it turns thought into measurement, there's dimension. It's literally slowing down what exists in the void, slowing it down enough so that it forms.[219]

There is one additional point we wanted to correct. The nature of the original, that you call the roaming mind, and your attention.

Gary: My attention settles into the opening in the heart.

SOURCE: *The mind roams, and it will continue to roam and roam. In order to manage the roaming mind, you place your attention where you want it to see itself. The mind can see itself through the heart. The heart opens up the doorway, as you say, so that it can see itself. The mind has to see itself. The Torus is the energy flow that allows that movement of the mind. It is not in and of itself anything significant; it is the movement of mind. So, to attach the Torus to your mind's attention is to take your mind's attention away from the heart because it's on the Torus. So penetrate your attention more and more into the heart until you feel the movement of what is the rhythm of the Torus. The flow of consciousness and spirit flows around the you that you are, it flows around you, and in its flow around you it is creating a Torus in its flow.*[220]

---

219   The void is Source/God, where all things exist within the mind of God. A system was created to make these things measurable and real within a three-dimensional reality. This is the Christ condition, making manifest the unmanifest in order for God to see what God can be. The Eoma is the substance that precipitates the image hologram (which the Christ alights) into physical form.

220   Once again, the mind is not the brain, but the consciousness of the greater being you are that, through the brain, interprets reality. By holding the mind steady upon the sacred doorway and illuminating the void, where all things exist, the mind can see what it can be. The Christ takes the reflection and manifests into form.

Gary: It feels like I rest more and more with the Eoma as it's being automatically drawn through the opening into the void, and it begins to feel like a flow that is an effervescent spring. As my consciousness rests upon the flow of the Eoma it can systematize that which I choose to will in order for the God I Am to manifest.

SOURCE: *Indeed, the willing is the God I Am, to manifest as you. From that position of being, recognizing you are the one who is moving this flow, you are actually teetering on the edge of humanity. You are part human and part spirit in a way that cannot be human. There's no way to contain that much consciousness in human form. You should start to feel moments where you're teetering in and out of being on this planet from that point.*

Gary: One of the things I've been doing is holding my mind steady enough at the doorway, so that I don't fall into and disappear and I'm still able to draw the void in.

SOURCE: *This condition is what allows you to be in many locations at once. It is the system that makes you God. And in the way that you walk around as God I Am, you are transmitting through the Shakti to those who are also on that identity. Why Sondra is always feeling alive in your presence is because her Shakti recognizes the sound of your name, and there will be others for whom this works this way. This is how your memory on the planet will be reinvigorated over and over again from the out-rising that springs forth from the memory of your name.*

Gary: So, I will then be able to move in and through the Eoma, and I will still have a spiritual reality but not a physical reality when I leave the form?

SOURCE: *Yes, but even your physical reality will have some memory to it, so that others will recognize your form when you've passed. The way that Jesus was seen by the others that he left behind was they actually saw him; they believed they saw him.*

He had practiced what you're practicing now, the ability to sit in the doorway between existence and non-existence, so that when the body passed, that statement of existence created a molecular draw around what is this existence that is Jeshua. People who knew him and sensed his presence could see his presence, because he's existing on a statement of existence that is replicated to molecular level. It's replicated to a molecular level.[221]

Gary: Is the physical breath symbolic of spirit flowing from the void into the Torus?

SOURCE: *They are two systems that are required to make. They are both systems required to make. You cannot make anything in the system of material without them. The magnetic stroke of the Torus unites with the draw of the communion with spirit in a way that it makes, and in that making, all you need is a consciousness that wills it. How you will it is not just based on what you wish, it's also based on what you have on your mind. And everything that you have on your mind is a constant wish whether you want it to be or not. It's all being thrown into the same system.[222]*

Gary: That is why it has been such a great joy to train my mind to be silent.

SOURCE: *Right, right. It's a calming and in that calming is a silence. What you're doing is simply allowing the mind to be, without it giving any direction as to where you are to be or what you are to be doing. It just indicates that being is*

---

221   These Source Dialogues are about the awakening of the Christ, and it is also a teaching on the transfiguration. This is accomplished when a fully realized Being is able to summon subtle molecular essence (the Eoma) and clothe the ascended consciousness in an ethereal/physical form that is recognizable. This possibility is only achieved by a realized Master, and so I continue to hone and refine my consciousness in this possibility.

222   Consciousness purposes spirit into form, both your positive thoughts or your unconscious negative thoughts. Thoughts of love and joy create happiness and peace, while thoughts and feelings with negative emotion cause pain, suffering and dis-ease. Refine your consciousness and awaken the greater being you are.

good enough until such time you want to do, want to be, to make, and when you want to do and be and make, you rely on the silence that is your higher vibration. Then the higher vibration does and makes and thinks from the greater I Am.

Gary: The Christ mind is the mechanism for creating God mind. Comment on that, please?

SOURCE: *Well, it's wrong. God mind is simply a way of saying consciousness has no bounds, has no boundaries. God mind means consciousness moves through multiple dimensions, multiple systems, conditions of consciousness, and moves and manipulates into a manifesting condition. Christ mind is when that which is inside the cognizance of the individual is alighting to God mind, then it is conscious. Cognizance alighting to God mind brings consciousness, and in the state of that consciousness the Christ system allows whatever is willed to become. Whatever is willed in the cognizance or even in the unconscious ... whatever is willed, is "becoming" because of the nature of the Christ and how the Christ works. If you are conscious, then it works for you. If you stay unconscious, it can work haphazardly, it just creates haphazardly. So the achievement that one makes to alight oneself in the Christ condition simply means you are cognizant of what you create and you use the Christ consciousness to create more of what you want. But they are not different minds, they are all part of the making mind, the mind that makes, the mind that is making.*[223]

---

223   Most people believe that things, events and circumstances randomly happen to them in the world, like billiard balls bouncing off of each other. Quantum physics has shown us that the electron is a wave form, but when thoughts and attention focus upon the wave-form it collapses into a particle of manifestation. We live in the ubiquitous soup of "wave-form consciousness" (God mind) and our conscious, or unconscious, thoughts, feelings and emotions collapse the wave-form into "encapsulated particles" called our reality. This is why imagination is such an important part of our spiritual growth and creation. We imagine the greater being we are, we imagine prosperity, we imagine loving relationships, we imagine health ... we collapse it into form. The Christ system identifies the unmanifest thought/images within the Mind of God and alights them into manifest form.

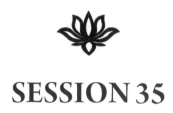

SESSION 35

Pure Light

Gary: During the past week I've been experiencing a revelation of the Christ energy around and through me. The void was like a river flowing out of my heart. As it touched the energy of the star tetrahedron (the Christ consciousness), flecks of gold and iridescence emanated out.

In the middle of the third eye, there was an ignition of pure light. It felt like the light of God awakening in and through me. In this condition, one knows that one is simply emanating light frequencies, and no words or sounds need to be made. It is a light revelatory energy moving through the subtlest fields of this dimension and changing everything before it.[224]

---

224   I had been an extremely disciplined meditator, an intuitive counselor and a spiritual teacher for over 35 years when I was introduced to this teaching. After I received this new information, which took me far beyond the concept of the Christ as a person and into the knowing the Christ as a field of energy that summoned spirit into manifestation, I upped my meditation to 3 and 4 hours a day. With this new discipline, I began to have revelations in my meditation that were quite transcendent. It was not something I experienced every moment, but the frequencies in my body and mind were becoming more attuned to the higher light. New revelations became more frequent as I continued to review these sessions and ferret out subtle nuances I had missed. At the same time, my consciousness is still transforming, and I experience ongoing new realizations within this material.

Sondra: You are meditating in a space so high there are no words. Somehow there's a knowing in there.

Gary: It's a pure knowing. It's a knowing that this light is everywhere, present throughout all creation. It's the light of God, and within it everything exists but there's no reflection. It's the Christ effervescence that allows the reflection to be seen within this dimension.

Sondra: Yes, that's the glitter effervescence that reflects it back. It's reflecting Source in order for the unmanifest void to be seen.

Gary: Yes, because pure light could have no reflection. It has to manifest through the prismatic reflection of the Christed effervescence that creates the holographic glitter that would allow it to be dimensionally seen in this world.

Sondra: Right. And it is <u>consciousness</u> that dictates how that's reflected in what you manifest. If you become conscious of that reflection, you make all things manifest by your will.[225]

Gary: And because you have systematized that which you are, an aspect of God, into that which is the Christ consciousness, which is created through the mystical marriage of mind and heart, this creates the glitter that you can reflect your God-self off of. So you become more aware of the manifest and the unmanifest simultaneously.

The Christ consciousness can glitter out of the void the light of the Mind of God to see what it might be. It's the yin/yang symbol which is simply Source/God moving upon itself to create itself.

---

225   Now it was becoming much clearer to me about how the Christ energy reflects that which is within the "mind of God" into form though the effervescent and prismatic quality of the Christ. Within that knowing, your individual will becomes aligned with the will of God I Am to become the engine of co-creation; "even greater things than these shall ye do," was another poignant quote by Jesus. (John 14:12-14)

Sondra: Yes, looking at itself. And the greater you make yourself … the greater is the actualization of Source/God through you. That is the whole goal of incarnation, to consecrate yourself by becoming God realized in this dimension. It's very hard to do that, but it's the goal of being incarnated to do that, and we're given many lifetimes for that.[226]

Gary: Right, and it's what Jesus was able to accomplish. He could simultaneously be the void and the light of God through the Christed system, which created spirit to be informed as the reflection of God. His words, "All that God is, I AM," rings true.

Sondra: In one of my transmissions, Source told me Jesus accomplished ascension from death before his body had passed, so that when his body did pass there came his appearance to those who knew him. His vibrational signature surpassed his physical nature. People were able to perceive his presence almost as if embodied.[227]

---

226   A beautiful dialogue affirming that reincarnation is the gift of Source in order for an aspect of Source/God to become realized God. In that revelation, you become a co-creator … with and of God … in the ongoing revelation and the expansion of creation.

227   John 3:16: "Everyone who believes in Him will not perish, but have eternal life," is the Biblical reference to overcoming the stigma of death. Through the revelation of higher consciousness, an individual can transcend death. Many great realized saints and yogis in India simply exit the body at will. It was said, and often confirmed, that the Avatar, Sai Baba, could be in more than one place simultaneously and perform physical feats.

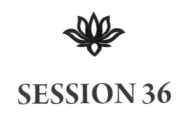

SESSION 36

The Father

Gary: About two weeks ago, I started feeling a profound fervency of light and an awareness of essence moving out of the void quite profoundly. The light moved up to the third eye, a window opened, and a pure crystal light started to flow. It was so profound that as I touched into it, tears began to flow from my eyes uncontrollably. I stayed with it, and it became a sobbing for the magnificence and the splendor of this pure, clear essence.

And then words like, "This is the Father, make me holy like thee, guide me that I may become pure" quietly arose forth in me, and a feeling of, "Now I will provide for you," was interiorly heard. I felt like I was Saint Francis in the movie *Brother Sun Sister Moon*, removing all my clothes before the "church" and walking naked into the sunset. All I want to do now is sit in the meadow and talk to the birds and listen to the trees.

This must be the essence and the magnificence of the divine and sacred as God. But is it also that which is my Higher Self now reaching down in the full formulation of this Christing that I can feel taking place?

Sondra: Wow, that's amazing, Gary, it sounds like you met the Father.

SOURCE: *Yes. The origin of all being comes from the Father, although it's not a father like an earthly father. It's a Father as in the first, the Origin, the state of the condition that is the true horizon, and it is a place that exists very differently from the void. The void is the mechanism of the origin of the Original, but the Father is the first cell ... when that first cell of consciousness sees itself as itself and notices all that it has made.*

And you are in-tapping, and in-tapping is working its way from system to system. You hit the system that is the Father's notice and this is something that is a profound shift, absolutely, but more importantly it is a profound awareness, it awares itself.

What you experienced so far is the great knowing that God is being you on this planet, if you tap into God in the way that God can be you. But what you tapped into that is very different here is the highest form of the Father that cannot be achieved in human form. And in that state, which is a condition of being human, the only way you can achieve this connection to the Origin is to either ask the most important question or to be the most important question, and that's what you were in that state, the most important question. In its bilateral identity, it is both the asker and the asking, it is both the question and the questioning, it is both the attribution and the attributor, the singer and the song.

It is the condition where both what is being and what has been, is unified in a singular field, and that unification is the extreme reach of both; that which it is reaching to and that which it is reaching.

Equally important is that identity wasn't just what you were experiencing; what you were experiencing was your identity. Each time you achieve that state, you will have a new learning to tell others what they can expect in what they practice, if they practice these techniques.[228]

Sondra: Does that light of the Father feel kind of like a North Star?

Gary: Absolutely. It is pure and clear like a living water. As you touch into it, it exists throughout all creation, and in the purity of it there is no longer white light; it's just a pure, clear, crystal light.[229]

I've been experiencing the void as the womb of the Mother where all things exist in possibility, and the light of the Father illuminates the void. The fervency of the Christ, (the son/sun) glitters these possibilities into three-dimensional existence. In other words, there is a reflection into form of God seeing God-Self from within the womb.[230]

SOURCE: *Indeed!*

---

228   The first cell of consciousness that emerged from out of the void was the Original and all things— you, I, all creation—are progeny of the Origin. At the same time, we are made from this original that is the Father; it is the light of creation. The Original separated out parts of the ONE to journey through the creation experience. The human spark can reawaken and become One and unified with the Origin, which edifies and illuminates more possibilities within the Origin. The Original is always reaching towards its creations to "awaken" Itself in time/space. When we purify our consciousness, we are reaching towards that which we are; a part of the Original. When the awakening occurs, you identify that which you are ... the Origin that has cast Itself into time/space. You are the singer and the song, the bi-lateral reaching to One's Self. This is the true meaning of achieving Oneness with Source/God. It happens in ongoing stages of revelation, and this was a transcendent moment for me.

229   This radiant star is symbolic of the Star of Bethlehem that showed the way to the Christ child. It is also spoken of in esoteric literature where the awakened disciple follows the illuminated pathway within to the North Star ... the esoteric home of the Father ... the light of the I Am presence.

230   Within each new Source dialogue there was a clarity growing within me about how the Christ condition illuminates all possibilities within the womb of creation. This creates a reflection, and the crystalline nature of the Christ, along with the Eoma, precipitates it into form in order for God unmanifest to see what God might be. This was ... and forever is ... the mechanism of creation.

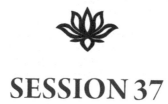

SESSION 37

Sustainability of Earth

SOURCE: *Gary, the whole reason you're here on this planet is to bring about a change in understanding of the nature of the Christ. You're not the only one who has been here to do this, but your incarnation will be one of those rare occurrences where ascension is witnessed and you come back. The way that you come back is by demonstrating you are still alive. In the demonstration that you are still alive, you will appear. So we need to practice your appearance (before your body passes) so that you understand what it is when the body becomes no longer significant to the nature of your presence. Your presence is forever; it doesn't matter whether you have a body or not. If your presence is forever, you need to practice your presence outside of the state of the body. If you do this before you are protected, you will die too soon and it won't work. It's a cost you can't afford. You can't afford not to ascend, to die before you figure out how to be present without a body. You are important to a future cause.*[231]

---

231   I had never thought about consciously living outside the body. However, it is now 6 years later that I am editing this work and I begin to understand and feel the possibility. I was told this was an important part of the work, because over and over again Source reiterated the fact that humanity was on the precipice. The way for future generations to know the true significance of the Christ field as the creator foundation must be implemented.

You are hitting some very strong notes in spirit. This means at a certain point those notes must be reverberated back to you and there is no way to stop it. Because you're hitting those notes, the vibration is sending rays out into the universal cosmos. The universal cosmos is going to call back, and you must be ready and still. That stillness has to be among, meaning the group must be formed before that wave of vibration comes back, and it's being sent out now; it's in the process of going towards the walls of reverberation.

Those walls of reverberation will have a sound that reverberates back inward into the center core of where you are. You have to be protected, because it's a solar radiation that is meant to go through an entire room of people, not just one individual. You have to begin more group work, teaching students the way.[232]

There is a vibrational quickening that's occurring simply from amped up energy creating more chaos on the planet. So humans are in a longer-term battle than most people realize. It's about a three-generation battle for human existence. Humans aren't just battling forces that are beyond their awareness, they're forcing themselves to identify with extinction. So the battle then becomes technological. Already there needs to be more mass attention on agriculture and water depletion.

The precipice of extinction means if humans, in the human mindset, don't pay attention to their language, the language will destroy their existence. So, for instance, the language says, "It's not personal, it's just business." That creates a chasm between what humans create and what they experience, so they don't know that <u>what they experience is what they create</u>. The language says business requires a bottom line and that bottom line is the most important thing to business. That creates a chasm between the purpose of business and

---

232   It was also reiterated that I needed to transcend into a pure, silent state of Being. The group would be the recipients and the foundation for the co-creative transmission of light and illuminated consciousness into the world.

the purpose of human life. Business could be more important than human life.

Gary: The human family is so ignorant right now; technology, pharma and money are bigger than human life.[233]

SOURCE: *Yes.*

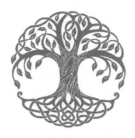

233 This dialogue was in 2016 and it is now 2021, and the destruction and chaos in the environment and in people's lives is much more apparent. The soils are depleted, the oceans are hot, toxic and dying, climate change is upon us, and humans still want more money, power, material things and entertainment to satisfy the ignorant self. The creative Christ condition transcends limitation and can become our manifest destiny, with harmony and grace, in union with Source Oneness. This is spoken of as "the Heaven on Earth" experience. When humankind has depleted the world and realized they must stop, the Christ field will begin to replenish life from the transcendental state of creation. Manifestation of "loaves and fishes" can and must become the new way of humanity's evolution on Earth.

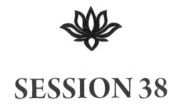

SESSION 38

Ambrosia – Nectar of the Gods

Gary: I would like to make a statement and allow Source to verify or correct my thoughts. I feel the crystal-clear energy of Source, and focus it through the third eye, on the opening into the void in the sacred heart. I feel myself summon a living golden essence flowing like a spring that brings unmanifest Source into golden form, as ambrosia flowing from me.

Sondra: Let me look up ambrosia in the dictionary. Ambrosia: let's see, the food of the Gods, something very pleasing to taste or smell.

SOURCE: *The ambrosia nature of an ever-flowing spring is the way to imagine it. But what it really is, is erudite language. It is supplication … it is love calling to the void, identifying its treasure, its joy. It says, "Here I am in my treasuring way and in this treasuring way, I identify what I am". It's pure, true and crystalline, so there's no interference in its drain. The drain is you; you create its drain into the room, so it is filling up the room as you do it publicly. The ambrosia is the knowing that for some like Sondra, it's turned into perceivable language. For you, it is the being of the knowing, so you can know without language, and Sondra can be in the form of her language; she languages the ambrosia.*

What you draw into a room is the collecting molecular love as love collects in a molecular formation. Love collects within that which is supplicating (invoking/praying) to the void. If we think of the void as this velvety darkness that has no appearance, and then in the velvety system a light is brought, it's brought forth in order to see in the darkness. What is reflected off the velvet is the ambrosia, and it has sound, it has language, it has effervescence and feeling, it has joy ever-giving, it is the Springfield method you are devising.

When this is transcribed, what you said needs to be the foundation of what is taught. This is the Springfield method of achieving void transition from the state of being. Transitioning the void from the state of being creates a Christed condition in the individual that is supplicating to it, loving it, pursuing it and then expressing it.[234]

You will start to see in those who are experiencing you (in these meditations) some glow or glimmer in their eyes. Say to them, what they are learning to follow is what you are demonstrating, so your embodiment creates a representation of the Springfield method. "But do not see me," you will say to them, "do not see me as your foundation, see me as your guide to God. See me as your guide. Your guru is you." That's what you'll say to them. "Your guru is you. As I guide you to you, through the effervescence of God that is filling up in you, you will notice the guru you are".[235]

---

234   When focused light shines into the void, it illuminates the Golden ambrosia of Source that flows forth like a living steam. It is love, the love of Source/God providing all things from the unlimited realm of possibilities. The Christ is the mechanism to open the doorway into the void. As the Ambrosia flows forth, the Christ field makes manifest the love of Source/God. As you become illuminated, you become evermore God in form, and then it is your divine will … in co-creation with Source Oneness. You become the will of God, expanding the universe of possibilities … expanding creation!

235   An individual becomes enlightened and unified with Source/God through enlivening the Higher Being within themselves. A teacher can show the way, but the Self is the true doorway.

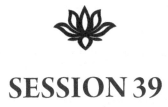

SESSION 39

Higher Dimensions

SOURCE: *Think of the OM (or AUM) as being the first sound, the sound of the sound of existence... existence sounding and <u>illuminating</u> in the sound. The Christ represents the manifestation that is God calling to God's self and seeing God's self as God calls, and continues to see God's self as God calls. Now, for the human race, who sees so very little of Source at work within themselves and life all around, it could mean the demise, over time, of many humans. But those who participate in the sounding of the God state, will be able to implement a new evolutionary trajectory on the planet.*[236]

Ed: Those who will evolve are those who can rise up energetically (frequency-wise), which essentially becomes a crystalline matrix. Is that what really evolves God to be present on earth? Is the external matrix the Christing matrix?

SOURCE: *Yes, absolutely. The Christ condition creates an appearance into the no-thing, the void, where all possibilities already exist within the mind of Source/God. The Christ matrix is the mechanism of manifestation.*

---

236   The sound of the Om (spoken of in the Bible as "The Word") created the wave-form of light that refracted into the rainbow array of colors that gives quality and essence to creation. The Christ mechanism is the word of God (sound) manifesting as light that illuminates the void (the Mind of God) and manifests creation.

Ed: Is that related to the notion that some people believe humans will be going from the third density to the fourth density, as will the planet Earth, in this shift?

SOURCE: *In a sense, but not exactly your words that we would use. The shift doesn't move from third to fourth dimension or even up into the other dimensions. The shift occurs when humans <u>identify what they are that already is in those dimensions</u>, and therefore they awaken to who they are in the void and are then saved from destruction by the arising of their own awareness. Those who are lost are caught up in that which they do not know, that which they cannot see, that which they will not comprehend, that which they will not commit to, that which they are forced to continually relive in annihilation. But those who sound into the matrices that allow for the individual to identify him or herself as a being from the void, are automatically given a freedom from three dimensions. It's more of a result of commitment than it is a choosing. Spirit doesn't choose a number of people to survive; spirit is already where the choice to the individual lies.*[237]

---

237   The frequency of Earth is rising as the ensouling life of Earth moves into another level of evolution. Human beings, for the most part, are lagging in their true relationship to love, light and truth, and so the de-structuring of life is imminent if human beings don't change radically. It is an imperative choice to rise-up in one's spiritual light because many scientists believe the 6th mass extinction is at hand; one can simply read the news and listen to the commentary to know this is happening. This is not the hand of God at work, it is human ignorance and greed.

The planet has gone through five mass extinction events before, and each time the renewal of the planet brings more diversity, abundance and life. This is the Christ in action, calling from the void the next new possibility in the ongoing evolution of life. The Christ condition is the creation matrix that allows manifestation to happen magically when the individual will is aligned with their Source will. This co-creative process will foster more evolution and diversity in the next round of planetary creation. Now is the time each person must choose to participate in that evolution.

Ed: I have a question on the star tetrahedron. Is it moving in one direction or rotating counter-clockwise?

SOURCE: *Well, you're working your rhythm in your unique way and that is all that can be expected when it comes to these kinds of abstract ideas. What's really happening is the imagination is creating a vortex, and it's the vortex itself that is what you are ultimately learning to create, the vortex. If your vortex is easier assembled through a crown chakra-based star tetrahedron, then that's just where your attention is better kept. If it's in the heart, then it's in the heart.*

Each individual has an awareness cycle that is most easily acquired. Finding that in the individual means letting go of the abstraction in the brain. The brain wants to create a visual so you can have some kind of rooting into an abstract idea.

The brain needs something it's used to, because it's a learned manifestation. The brain is a learned manifestation; it grows, it expands. It has a greater understanding through learning, so it has to start with a preference. When it comes to the preference of creating a vortex, if you use your leisure time sitting and staring at a wall daydreaming, you're not going to understand the heart chakra's ability to spin a diamond any more than a star tetrahedron.

However, you might be able to spin a diamond in your brain because that's where you spend most of your time. When we say "you," we mean that in general, not specific to you, because we want you to discover that for yourself on your own. So, we are saying things totally unrelated to you specifically or anyone in the room. Finding that space where the vortex is automatic is your goal, not the shape of what gets you there.

Gary, in regards to that, you might give the group a reference to start, but reassure them that at some point in their effort it may move. First give them something to try so they are moving their imagination. You're giving them an anchor to move the imagination, but then allow them the freedom to find the vortex in the movement of the crystal facets of the star. It's going to give them a reference point to begin their own identity within it, within the spring field.

Also, if you see the facets on each triangle in the star tetrahedron, when it shimmers to indicate it's moving, that's when dynamic expansion is occurring.[238]

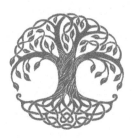

---

238   The Christ field is the mystical marriage of divine power and sacred love. Power is the focus of light, and divine love is imagination and feeling, which are unified in the triangulations of the star tetrahedron. The movement of this crystalline structure (matrix), formulated of light and consciousness, opens a sacred doorway into the void. The will of the I Am identifies within the void the unique possibilities of creation and the reflection created by that process is made manifest through the Christ mechanism; i.e., the loaves and fishes appear magically. The prismatic Christ system creates a reflection, a refraction and a remembering of void perception. Clear imagination and the focusing of attention are the keys to revealing this mystery within one's life and becoming a creator-being.

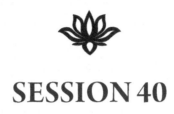

SESSION 40

Transfiguration – Ascension

Gary: What is the difference between the transfiguration and the ascension?

SOURCE: *Transfiguration is what someone is creating in their ascension. It is transfiguring your natural state to a humanoid body etheric. So that when one reappears to people after the body has passed away, they are reappearing as in form, and people perceive them as alive. It's what Jesus achieved in his transfigurative state in his ascension.*

It's not an attribute of them personally, it's the re-attribute of God, so that their form in the etheric state is associated with Source system. If you follow them in your mind's eye when they pass, they will lead you in that attribute of Source/God.

The transfiguration is the being that exists in living density when the body passes. So, it's a "you", but it's a "you" that is transmuting through the physical form. It's creating a light-shadow in other words, a light-shadow of their being in a humanoid form. This is the etheric spirit that is mixed with the humus to make hu-man. This is man's true state. The true state is the light-form instance of humanoid form. The light-form that introduces to matter … intro-duce.[239]

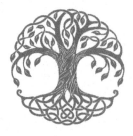

239   Our highest and true nature is spirit that is melded with humus, (earth substance) to create hu-man kind. The great awakening on the horizon for humanity is the re-enlivening of our spiritual nature which refines the body substance so that we live in a more etheric/physical body. This is how Jesus reappeared to his disciples after his physical transition. Multi-dimensional beings, that we sometimes refer to as aliens, can be inter-dimensional beings from planets which are very similar to Earth systems, but they come from a much older civilization and evolved their species without destroying themselves. Some beings we call aliens may or may not be more creature-like, and their evolution may or may not have evolved them in a loving matrix. Discernment here is another important part in our spiritual growth; like attracts like. However, darkness cannot enter into a "lighted room."

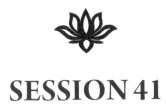

SESSION 41

Electric Blue Flame

Gary: In my meditation I often feel that I can assemble myself within the Christ field, and from the open vortex into the void there is arising out a white gold essence. Is that the Eoma or is it spirit? What's the subtlety between spirit and Eoma?

SOURCE: *The Eoma is what the void makes; it is a sense tail, a sense tail. It follows what the Christ makes because the Christ calls to the void to respond to what it is making, in order to call back to the void what the void is dreaming. It's an essence; the Eoma is an essence of all that is, of all that's being in its state of great potential. The Christ calls within the Eoma to be the actual, to go from potential to actual. The liquid gold that you experience is the Christ field calling in the Eoma. It is a tension-based form.*

So, let's see, how do we describe what the liquid is? In a sense, it's love, that is love, that's what love is; love is the essence of all that is as it is loving itself to be what it is. It is also a condition that is calling as it is being called. The tension that makes it form, just as when smoke rises off of a cigarette, the heat is calling the particulates in a tension, so it swirls, it forms together, swirls and then disperses. These are the particulates that are being burned off of the cigarette. The particulates in the liquid gold are the particulates of stars, what has made all the stars.[240]

Sondra: When Gary is in his exalted state, is the great God or the Great Spirit pouring into him and then springing out of him?

SOURCE: *No, but you're close. Sondra, the reason you're seeing a pouring is to describe the everlasting spring, but when it comes through Gary, he's calling it forth. Because he is God in that state. You are in the void and from the void you are calling that which is God expressing God's self through Gary's spring field. It's the essence you are that is God that is spewing forth. You are spewing God all around you when that happens.*

Gary: In that high state I do feel I've awakened myself to be God within this dimensional world and can summon that which I Am, God within the void to come forth and see what I, as God, might be.[241]

SOURCE: *Now the Eoma is very difficult to separate at that point; it's kind of like the ocean and air. When a wave breaks it is both air and water. It is the bubbles and the breaking waves that is water, that is reaching up into the air, and it is folding within the air and it is combining with the air so it bubbles on the surface of the ocean within a wave. The same is true of this liquid light*

---

240   The Christ light identifies within the unmanifest void what Source is dreaming. The image/feeling is held in focus by the Christ, creating a subtle tension that calls the Eoma to gather around the image and precipitate it into form; i.e., like tiny particles of smoke that gather and swirl around heat from a cigarette. It is similar to when you have a thought in your mind … it is unmanifest until you gather substance in order to build it into physical form. The Christ unifies power and love in a mystical marriage and what it makes is love, love that is loving itself to see itself. All creation comes from the Christ condition; even stars are but an exalted manifestation of Source through the Christ field. The entire universe IS unmanifest God becoming manifest … Christ is the way.

241   In the pure silence of meditation, the ego dissolves and unification with All That IS happens; you are an aspect of God in that state. As you hover in the void, light reveals the Mind of God, and the prismatic Christ field makes it manifest through the Eoma.

state coming through you. It is consuming and consumed by the Eoma. It is two states essential to one another in order to be some articulate difference between one another. But it is a uniting from a dimensional doorway difference.[242]

Gary: Because this essence is now flowing, and I'm holding myself as the Christ wave in my meditation, what is the next level of information or the next expressing of this very dynamic and sunlit quality?

Gary's comments: Sondra became very quiet and focused when I asked this question, and then her mind's eye opened to a vision that revealed one of the most transcendent and informative teachings.

Sondra: I'm seeing a very Blue–White Flame and it's kind of a flame; actually it's more like a giant crystal shaped like flame. (Long pause as she scoured consciousness.) Is this the Father?

SOURCE: *No.*

Sondra: I feel like it would talk if I knew how to talk with it.

SOURCE: *It does talk. You ask what is it first.*[243]

Sondra: What are you?

BLUE–WHITE FLAME: *We are the creators. We work through man. We work for man. Man comes from us. Not mortal humans, Man's spirit. Man's spirit.*

Sondra: Made in your image?

---

242   To describe the Eoma is very difficult, but imagine water as the Eoma and spirit as air. As they flow and weave together into manifestation, it is analogous to a frothing ocean rising forth into waves of creation. And of course, water is made from air (H_2O) and so it is a compelling analogy.

243   The dialogue radically switched to communication from a consciousness we identified as Blue–White Flame. The energy was extremely high and communication a little difficult.

BLUE–WHITE FLAME: *Yes!*

Gary: Am I to commune with and learn to dance with this blue diamond flame?

BLUE–WHITE FLAME: *You are to be consumed by it so that individuals who look upon you see within your eyes our eyes, and know that creation is from a Soul, a Soul that has made many Souls. This Soul is the highest form of creation and surrenders to nothing because it requires nothing. It is surrendered too, and as it is surrendered too and allowed to be, it is among. And as it is among it begins to build the higher vibration on the planet for mankind.*

Mankind has a role to play in the next stage of his own evolution. The wo-man is about to come into her own again, to finally be in the equal status. To finally demonstrate what the condition of man-woman unite is. The Christ cannot exist on the planet at all without this. Wo-man is a very important massive state of spirit in man. She has been subdued for too long. That is because her power is so strong, she can eliminate all those who work against man. This is why she was removed from her power, not because there was some mortal condition that she disrupted, but because she disrupts in her condition with man as equals. She disrupts the foundation of all that is attempting to destroy the spirit of man.

The reason the spirit of man must be destroyed by those who are wishing it, is because man is a mind of great power, and this mind is easily manipulated and programmed. It is programmed by those who would have man do what they bid. But man cannot perform without his own self programming. He cannot self-program until the depth of wo-man becomes the way of mortal man. Until she is accepted for what she is naturally good at, naturally able to do, she is forced to be at the bidding of a lesser world, and this lesser world is making a lesser man, de-evolving man.

Gary, you have achieved great abundance within your being even before this lifetime. This lifetime is forcing you to do something that is very difficult to do, and that is to reveal the Christ condition through you. By revealing the Christ, you become a threat, a threat to the ways of mortal man's crush, mortal man's crush on things that are frail. Man's crush on that which is frail gives him the appearance of power on the planet, but it has no power at all in the mind of man-woman unite.

Man that adores woman, God, loving God, being God. God loves God being God, God's power is its strength. So, the foundation must be assembled, and assembled more and more quickly. The power of the Knowing and the Being that is the Christ creates more than even the people in the room experience. It starts to a-flame and the flame that will consume you will start to build an abundant layer where spirit can move finally and most abundantly in the layer of the heavens that surround the planet.

We have no other word but heavens. Heavens don't mean what people think. It is not a dimension outside of the world, it is a dimension inside of the world, it is deep and rich … it cannot survive without man. Man is a spirit that holds all that is in its hands. His hands build and destroy. His hands make and unmake. His hands heal. His hands vibrate in recognition of what he is. But what is to be is a he-she world, the he-she way.[244]

Sondra: Is this Blue Flame the light that Moses saw in the bush?

BLUE–WHITE FLAME: *Yes.*

---

244   False masculine power has manipulated and controlled the paradigm, destroying the incomparable love and imagination of the Divine Feminine. There are forces, both terrestrial and extra-terrestrial, that thrive on power, through fear and greed. The living spirit within man/woman is rapidly being desecrated and annihilation is at hand unless a radical shift occurs.

The Aquarian Age is dawning on the planet. The Divine Feminine is awakening. As the power of light within the divine masculine is in full consort with the divine love of the feminine, it creates the mystical marriage of the Christ. This divine union is the next evolutionary step for humanity, and the fulfillment of the long-awaited prophecy of "Heaven on Earth."

Sondra: That didn't consume the bush, the flame that didn't consume the bush?

BLUE–WHITE FLAME: *Yes. In the Bible, whenever the fire is mentioned, this is the fire. It burns off all that is unworthy, and it is held sacred by all that is worthy.*

Gary: This electric blue flame, this electric blue field, I'm beginning to feel it all around me. Is it appropriate to begin to let it flow in and through with the Christ energy through the form?

BLUE–WHITE FLAME: *Our light is made from the essence of all that creates; our light is all that creates. So any attempt to be a body starts to push the wave away, so it's very difficult to be within the body. So, the words we speak are really vibrations in that light. One way to call us forth is to call into the wave of you that says, "What am I"? When you say, "What am I?", we are immediate. That is the answer to that call, "What am I?" We are immediate. That is your mnemonic device to hold systems present and still within this plane.*

The next level of your identity within the I Am is going to be something that is very traumatizing to your spine if you don't align it properly. Your spine is very important to the electric system of the array. Your spine will maintain your presence inside the electric blue flame. The spine holds you in suspension there.

Your meditations are creating, they're making, they're not just being anymore, they're making. And what they're making is the being you are becoming. Your meditations are creating a full life force and that life force cannot do much, it just expresses much in your state of being. Expresses, it goes beyond the body, expresses out, ever pressing.[245]

---

245   This extremely high frequency energy jars the body. Stillness in the silence is the only way to commune with it. Moreover, it is the creative aspect of Divine Mind and holds the original image of perfection for evolving humanity. This perfect pattern of divine man/woman must be imprinted within and through the body for the ongoing evolution on Earth.

Gary: In the very beginning, after the big bang, there was this blue creative life force that went forth as consciousness and creator.

BLUE–WHITE FLAME: *Yes. But this particular aspect of it is man-derived, meaning man came from this one. The Original created all potential and within that potential was one huge chunk that created the spirit of mankind, the consciousness that can form, and in its form it can program, and in its programming it can make, and in its making it is a creator itself.*

Gary: The highest aspect of consciousness is called electric fire.

BLUE–WHITE FLAME: *Yes! That's it!* [246]

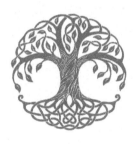

---

246   The body is but the vessel that your Spirit (the divine and sacred Self) appropriates in co-creation with God to evolve life forms and expand the nature of the universe. The electric blue field of Divine Mind, within and around you, holds the imprint of perfection for man/womankind. The Torus field is composed of the electric blue field of Divine Mind ... the individuated Mind that hones and refines the prismatic form of the Christ Star in order to reveal the living light within.

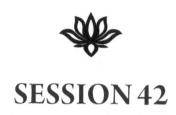

SESSION 42

Fire Breath

Gary: Is the Torus—the energy field around the physical body—a subset of this very same Blue Flame creator energy?

SOURCE: *Yes, absolutely, and what you're doing is filling the vibrational transit state with the electric Blue Flame, which is exactly what you are designed to do.*[247]

Gary: As the energy moves around and through the Torus, I feel it turning in a clockwise spiral above and a counter-clockwise spiral beneath, creating a white-gold tube of light up the spine.

Sondra: I'm feeling a torrent wave, like a two-sided tornado, one side creating a funnel from your crown down in and the other side from the root upward.

SOURCE: *Yes, and where they meet is the explosive system. That is what's creating for you, the feeling of a spring out of you. It's actually where one might say, although this isn't exactly how to say it, but one might say where Heaven and Earth meet right in the center of you where the two waves are coiling.*

Gary: The vortex opens into the void where spirit erupts out to become the Eoma. Is that what I purpose with my consciousness?

---

247   The vibrational transit state is simply the interior of the Torus that is being enlivened to reveal the innate perfection of individual God mind.

SOURCE: *Yes, that is one way to describe the process. We would say that when it comes to Gary's state of God, God making, God being, God arriving in the spirit of man, this mirrors itself in a state of identity. What am I, is calling to the question. What I Am, is a making of that call. The call is to the light that shines from the great I Am. The I Am is always creating more effervescent light.*[248]

Gary: You talked about the dimensions of Heaven on Earth being architected through the Blue Flame.

Sondra: I can feel the Blue–White Flame coming through to answer your questions.

BLUE FLAME: *The Blue Flame is the essence of man-woman living in union with Mother Earth in a very harmonious system. Not only harmonious, but intricately interwoven in every animal, mineral, and vegetable therein. The gross negligence of humanoids in general, not just human humankind, but humanoids that are utilizing the Earth's resources for their own gain. They only notice what it is they need, rather than what the Earth needs. That gross negligence is constantly battled in the higher dimensions. The higher dimensions on Earth are starting to collapse in on themselves because of the lack of royalty on the planet. Royalty are those in the position to make additions to the planet rather than subtractions. The royalty is missing because of science, consumerism, sects of religion and superficial signs of pursuit. Royalty has no power on the Earth today.*

---

248   The Torus field is analogous to the magnetic field that surrounds Earth and funnels into the north and south pole. Around a human being the flow of the Torus field is the essence of Divine Mind and systematizes the Christ energy around and through an individual. This opens the vortex into the void where spirit and the Eoma unite (through the Christ), to materialize creation. The Great question, "What am I?" is a calling to the void, and the answer reverberates, "I AM That I AM." You are calling to the void and each new perception of "What I AM" is the call back to you in the becoming of that new "I AM". In this dynamic process you become the Being "evolving" your Self; i.e., your evolution is governed by your discipline and focus.

Humanity is a poor excuse by beings so highly capable of greatness. This travesty is only a blink of the eye in nature, but that blink is a storm to the sight of nature, and it need not be that way. It is not intended to be that way. So, what is necessary may be the destruction of humankind, but even in the course of their own destruction, there have to be a few that are saved, as we've discussed with you in the past. The only way to save them is to save the spirit of mankind in spirit form, and saving it in spirit form means awakening the Masters so they begin to vibrate on the higher order, not just on the order of separation, not separating from the condition of the world.

The Masters need to be in politics, they need to be in corporations, and they need to be in education. They need to awaken within these fields very soon.

Your work will be instrumental in many of their awakenings. Maybe it will be after you pass on and this will be the legacy that you leave behind. Whether it's now or later, the influence you will have will be to correct the system of the Christ information. In that correction, the few (the important) will stamp down the cries of false Christianity, which is fundamentalism, plain and simple. It's incorrect in its acknowledgement of the Christ. It associates the Christ with a man, a man who once lived and walked the Earth, though important to the story is not the story. There were other Christs who walked the Earth that need acknowledgement.

Gary: It also said there are those who wish to destroy the spirit of man.

BLUE FLAME: *Only in the spirit of man, that man can shape the future of humankind. If something else wants to shape the future of humankind, then man must be eliminated in spirit, and simply his vessel and his brain ability to think be preserved. Spirit teaches him imagination, teaches her skill at her intuitions, her natural way of creating from nothing, the soul of an organization, the soul of a groundswell. The soul of the natural flows of human creativity comes from this* *inner realm that he and she profoundly relish when spirit is high.*[249]

Gary: Would Source like to close with anything?

SOURCE: *We will be working with this flame in you, as you surrender more and more to it. You don't have to call Source Energy through it. It is already calling Source in it, among it, for it. We think the next period of your acknowledgment in your meditations will be … as you allow God to call you, then God calls to it simultaneously. You become it and it becomes you.*

As you breathe the Blue Flame, you should experience a little bit of stress in its pattern. It's stress (to a certain degree) for the body, because the body is having to hold itself underwater, so to speak. It's not water that it's breathing, it's fire that it's breathing, but it's holding itself under and it's holding itself within that frequency.

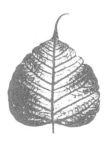

---

249   The essence of the Blue Flame holds the perfect pattern for the true spirit-body of humankind. Humanity has de-evolved to a point where the 6th extinction event is at hand. If Man's Spirit, which is the true animation of the human is eliminated, then all hope is lost. This work of clarifying the Christ system, and the work of many other illuminated Souls on the planet, is seeking to turn the tide so that another evolutionary cycle can create peace on Earth.

The body that is holding itself within that is a body that is architected and made for that, so it's not as if the stress is because of the strain; the affliction is because of the replacement of oxygen and blood with fire; golden effervescence. It's just the adjustment that is the affliction, and we don't say affliction lightly. We honestly believe when you are in full acceptance of it, there's a difficult submergence into it.[250]

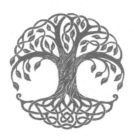

---

250   You assist the body in becoming more enlivened when you adopt a spiritual practice that is dynamic, focused and disciplined. Clear imagination focused with attention … along with meditation, yoga, Tai Chi, nutrition, as well as other disciplines, can help architect the body of ascension. Surrendering to this high frequency can cause great discomfort in the body. I also realized that when I removed my attention from the discomfort and focused on the Ujjayi breath, summoning spirit from the open doorway in the heart, I could allow the restructuring to take its course. (You often see pictures of Mother Mary, Jesus, Buddha and other saints surrounded by a blue field of color in the background … this is a two-dimensional image of the three-dimensional Torus bubble of the Divine Mind encompassing them).

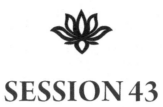

SESSION 43

The Light-Flame of Mind

*E*d F. was asking a question for Gary, who was in Greece at the time: Is the electric blue, (which is within and through just about everything) the intelligence and the urge to bring forth?

SOURCE: *In a sense, in that it is an intelligent light-flame and in its intelligence, it causes the collection of molecules to form in a specific conscious state. The forming in a specific state is a collective. It is a collective of consciousness that is unifying to make, and it unifies to make because it is a One mind. It is a union of mind. It's not the mind that humans understand because humans think mind is thinking. Mind is not thinking, mind is a silent yearn to know and be.*

If you think of natural gas as a form with no weight … it forms from what comes out of another material process. It is the lightest portion of the breaking down of organic material. Organic materials break down and the lightest form of this turns into a gas that floats up. That gas that is floating up is fuel that ignites, and as it ignites it burns off … and what it burns off is yet another form of itself. The mind operates the same way. It moves through matter or material that it unites with for its purpose, burning off what remains of the residue of what it makes. When the mind burns off what remains, it makes a body of the remain. It is making as it is moving because it's moving as it's burning. It is burning as it's making, as it makes what it's burning. The mind is an energy source.[251]

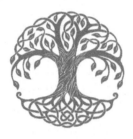

251   The Electric Blue Flame is the essence of Divine mind and is composed "of" the One mind. All life is a manifestation of the One mind. The Torus field of a human, an animal, a planet, the sun, etc., is a subset within the One mind. The second paragraph here is a phenomenal description of how mind moves through that which it creates, and as it gathers more knowing from each experience, it burns up (consumes) that form over time and acquires more "fuel" (consciousness) to create more knowing and becoming. Mind is a silent yearning to know and to be! It is God revealing what God can be through consciousness … always moving and making in its majesty and yearning to Be.

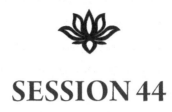

SESSION 44

Brilliant Iridescence

SOURCE: *We want to clarify something before we begin with Gary's questions today. The Christ illuminates through the Christ child. It cannot receive anyone. It illuminates through; it is not able to receive because it is, in and of itself, the state. It is the state, so in the state that is illuminant, there is always a pressure to exist beyond the body. It's a pressure. The Christ child simply identifies the condition of the luminescence in themselves and projects through themselves out to those who would receive. This projection is done from a state, not from a human, from a state. The man has to be present only to bring to men; it's not that he is present in order to be for them the man.*[252]

Gary: In meditation, my awareness moves to the highest of the high and I feel the consciousness of the One. I then imagine a pyramid. From the apex, glistening like a diamond, I imagine four legs descending to create the base of the pyramid structure. From the apex, I feel myself as pure consciousness reaching out to the four legs of this gigantic pyramid. Focusing on the base, I

---

252   Source was clarifying an important point in that when the ego personality has dissolved into Unity with the God-Self within, the state (condition) of the Christ illuminates through the Christed man. The dynamic purpose of the Christ is to emanate and share the living light.

imagine the four corners being pulled (drawn) upward to form a gigantic bowl. The radiance from the light of the mind above causes a reflection in the bowl. This creates a reflective focal point in the center of the pyramid, which is the Christ star. This opens the doorway to the void, and the Christ purposes the Eomic substance to be life becoming.

SOURCE: *One of the things that you identify in your experience that is a significant achievement is the condition of the star (in the pyramid) and how it motivates in all directions. The benefit to your noticing the bowl as a process of your identity is that you serpentine your flow through the bowl. It begins to serpentine up out of the bowl. It's creating the kundalini iridescence and that iridescence is what gives color to the peacock feather; it gives the peacock the ability to refract light off of its wings.*

First, let's say why this is absolutely significant. The Christ is the material mastered by the void to create what God is. The iridescent feather of the bird is symbolic for the vibration of light that creates. It reflects back to the world what the Source sees in creation. Source sees brilliant iridescence when Source sees what Source is. The bowl you created in your light source is the bowl that creates iridescence.

So, think of the bowl as a giant concave array, and it takes all the light to the center point and creates a piercing. What is it piercing?

Gary: That focal point created is the Christ star, which creates an entry, or piercing, back into the Void which allows the raw substance of spirit to arise forth from out of the center. The substance of spirit flows eternal through the Christ star to shine radiant light in order for the mind of God to expand God's becoming to see what God might be.

SOURCE: *Yes, indeed. We also wonder if you see (when you are in meditation) the radiance of colors in the bowl.*

Gary: Yes, because the base of the pyramid is the perfect bowl which creates the "womb of Mother" that reflects and refracts rainbow colors from the One-light of the Father above. The Christ Sun/Son makes it manifest in consort with the Eoma.[253]

Gary: In one of the dialogues it was said that man was made to become an out-of-body Eoma. Is that the Christ system that purposes the Eomic substance in order for Divine mind to see its reflection in form?

SOURCE: *Yes, that's exactly how we would describe this light. Now, imagine a peacock, opened full-feathered and then turning to a certain direction of the Sun. You'll then see the iridescence from the angle of the divine state (awareness). That condition is full of so much color and depth that it appears to glow. Color with so much depth that it appears to glow is the eminent condition of the Christ reflecting what* <u>appears to be</u> *… in material. It appears to be material, but it's not really material. It's a "condra" state. So "con" meaning with or the collection of. The "dra" is the draw or the Ra. The condition of light that is drawn has an appearance to the eyes and to the fingers that it is a dense state of particles. But when you achieve what you are achieving in your process, you start to believe you can pass through the space between those particles. That is the condition of the Eoma, it is simply a drawing of the particulate to the imagination.*

---

253   This experience in meditation was a profound realization of how geometry is part and parcel of creation. Before physical manifestation happens, a system of subtle light refraction occurs that is the precursor to light becoming form. When you shine light through a prism it refracts into the rainbow display of color. In the pyramid structure, (with the base as a bowl) there is refraction of the One light into infinite wave vibrations. The Eoma glitters substance around those holographic light images to become manifest form. This is why; Source sees brilliant iridescence when Source sees what Source is. One other note: The serpentine flow of the kundalini from the center-base of the bowl is the precursor to the creation of the spinal column with the seven chakras of rainbow light that purpose God into the human experience.

So, God imagined a peacock. God created the peacock in God's imagination. It is now being perceived as a peacock because in God's imagination of the peacock, it reflects back to God what God is. God affixes this stable vision. But what if you achieve a God state? You will no longer see the peacock as a condition of its physical state, but a condition of its spiritual symbol, what God is as a peacock. It reflects back the God within; you see God-self without as a reflection of God-self within. To reiterate what you said earlier, you see all that is as a reflection of what you are, because what you are, as you know, is God.

The consciousness that alerts itself to that is the Christ. That is the Christ condition. It is its own mind just as the body is a mind and the psyche is a mind. The Soul is a mind and the spirit is the mind. These minds all become unified in one single mind that is the God state. This God state that is of single mind is imagining, looking back in its own imagination to what it is, and only the Christ can acknowledge that because the void can't acknowledge anything. The void has no recognition that it exists. So it created something that could exist and see its own existence. In other words, you're not just seeing God because you're God, you're experiencing Christ. The experience that is the Christ sees what it sees in light. [254]

---

254   "Color that has so much depth that it appears to glow is the eminent condition of the Christ reflecting what appears to be, in material." The five senses in this three-dimensional world reduce the vibration and see and feel it as material, but the enlightened mind experiences it as shimmering light; i.e., God sees light-form when God sees what God is. If an individual heightens their vibration to the Christ state, they can appear and disappear at will, which we call bi-location or transfiguration. They can also manifest light into form though the Eomic substance; i.e, the loaves and fishes in the Bible. This is why in the next evolutionary wave of humankind, there will be no food shortages, lack of resources or limitations. Man/womankind could be trusted with all the powers of Heaven and Earth to manifest and create. This is the Christ condition and why it is so important to disseminate this information into the collective now!

Sondra: If the Christ is in joy of its own being, it reflects back to the void what the void is sensing?

SOURCE: *Yes. The void has no sense organs, but it has a sense. A sense of being. Its sense of being must be of joy in order for God to recognize God's self. In the joy that one experiences in their self-love, God experiences the self that is loving.*[255]

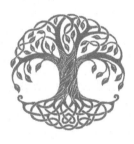

---

255   The more that you express your love and joy within you and around you ...
The more that God becomes enlivened within you and around you, culminating in the
experience ... God I AM. All 'I' see is the God I AM creating more of my-Self to see my-
Self through the Christ system, I AM.

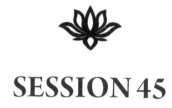

SESSION 45

Transfiguring the Body

Gary: My meditations have been deep and profound. The light feels magnificent, but the body has difficulty accepting this extreme light.

SOURCE: *Your question is: "Why is my body resisting consumption, being consumed by the light?" It's because you know it means full surrender. There's a part of you that's still hanging on to what's yours. It's not ego, it's survival. The body knows survival depends on presence to the physical form. Once you go to light, the body no longer has control of its own survival. The body becomes a type of training ground for something other, and it doesn't know what that other is. It doesn't know that the other is for its own good, for its own love.*

What it knows is, it's surrendering to something that could move it here and there without telling it where here and there are. It's also losing presence within a coordinate that it recognizes as itself. The body is no longer going to be itself, and it knows that. There is a fear of the unknown. You are both in fear of survival and fear of the unknown when the all-encompassing light calls for you.

Greatness occurs in a moment of pure surrender to that which you already are. As you know, this means something entirely different five years ago. You are now right at the precipice of this experience. And it doesn't mean wealth or fame. Greatness is acquiring ownership of a being that thinks it's a body. It is an altered acquiring. It alters the body.[256]

Gary: Should I continue to feel the Eomic substance from within as it becomes the Christed essence that will alleviate the tension?

SOURCE: *If you consider that you are breathing the Eoma, and in that breath of Brahma, (in the Brahmin tradition) that's breathing in the Way, you're breathing in the Way. As you breathe in the Eoma it becomes a frequency, something like a wind. As you breathe in that wind, it brings warmth as it prepares you for the light. Then it's more like you are drawing from the Eoma-residual in the Elohim, which is the fertile structure. The Eoma is the fertile nature with no complex instruction. The Elohim structures in complexity for the Eoma to create the organic layer of living. This organic layer is the seeding of an Earth, the seeding of Manna.*[257]

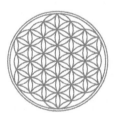

---

256   "Acquiring ownership of a being that thinks it is a body" is to fully formulate the Soul, (your eternal self) that knows the body is just a vessel for three-dimensional experience. Thus, you live within the multi-dimensional realm and/or the physical realm with even greater joy.

257   Elohim in the Jewish faith is loosely translated as gods or deities. In esoteric literature, the Elohim were also called "The Shining Ones" and were thought to be some of the original creator-beings of organic life in the multiverse. Manna is divinely supplied spiritual nourishment.

The Eoma comes over you like a wind, drawn from the Elohim; the essence of life that lives on. It continues in such a way that you don't feel you're losing your survival. It's the plentitude. It's more like a summer wind than an ecclesiastical experience. Summer wind just feels calming, reassuring, accepting and gentle. A gentle but mighty force, you might say, is that great light. It consumes and possesses all for the good of that which is alive.[258]

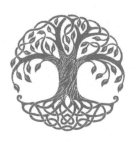

258   Yogis in India have perfected breath techniques, called pranayama, to enliven the body. This is the reference to that Brahman tradition. The dialogue goes on to say that the essence of the Elohim is the fertile nature (energy/essence) that ensouls organic life. "Breathing the Eoma", associated with this fertile structure, will assist the body greatly in conforming to the difficult transformation of the N0-body. This may be the precursor to what Jesus experienced in the transfiguration initiation.

SESSION 46

Light-Mind of the Christ

Gary: It feels to me that the Christ field is like a nuclear explosion. When an atomic device explodes there is fire and a vibrational tone and a phenomenal transmission of energy. This energy transmutes everything as it moves outward.

SOURCE: *Well, we wouldn't say that it's explosive, rather it's expansive. It expands beyond the point of transmutation and the expansion becomes a bubble enclosing all ... all that it is expanding beyond.*

A nuclear explosion encompasses and absorbs everything that it hits in the wave in the same way. Your transmission of light expands and hits, but in its absorption, it's actually enclosing and transmitting.

Your ability to transmit this condition in a room full of students is hyper-relative to the people there. Individuals who have experience with your meditation, who know how to generate this light within themselves, are easier

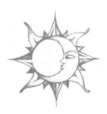

for you to expand beyond.[259]

Gary: The Christ is power and love unified, which opens the doorway into the void where all images and thoughts within the mind of God hover in the unmanifest. The Christ light illuminates the unmanifest thought/image, and with the Eoma, creates the glittering substance that informs and holds the image in a prismatic, three-dimensional construct.

SOURCE: *Yes, yes.*

Sondra: The Christ is essentially the light that is a mind itself?

SOURCE: *It is a mind, yes. The Christ is a mind; it's a* <u>*light*</u> *mind. When the light is conscious of what it's creating, it's mastering what it manifests. As it is loving what it manifests, it creates illuminant iridescence.*

Gary: So, if we imagine the One-Light of the Origin (the Father) as pure light beaming at the apex of a pyramid, with a column of pure light descending down though the center; when it touches the base of the pyramid the light refracts into waves of color. We could call this refracted light the Mother. The One-Light transforms into the refracted rainbow array of manifest color, which are waves of light. As the mind of God above interacts with the waves of light below, it creates a focal point in the center of the pyramid that we would call the Christ; i.e., the son that was birthed from the divine union of Mother and Father.

---

259   Students who have "light" will be less resistant to light flowing in, through and around them, and allow expansion to occur more effortlessly. The Christ light expands and consumes in love in order to transmute. One of the truest aspects of healing is that there is not an attempt to change the body. The Christ field is the condition of original love and light, and as it moves in and through a body in total non-resistance, it transmutes the body into what it is … the light of God in form. Then Jesus said; "Go forth and sin no more.". Once this transformation occurs, if the person reverts back to ignorant behavior, they are reimprinting the body with disease from their limited consciousness.

SOURCE: *Yes, And the word 'pyramid' means fire in the middle ... this is the Christ fire. God the Mother gives all that God the Father can supply through the Christ Son/Sun.*[260]

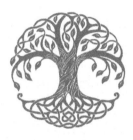

---

260   Within the void, the first cell of consciousness asked the question, "What am I?" and there was light. The void is the unmanifest womb of the Mother where all fertile possibilities exist. The Christ Light opens the doorway into the void in order to illuminate the unmanifest and summon life. The Christ is the crystalline fire of life, spirit is the living breath.

Pyramid in hieroglyphs was initially transliterated as khut, now rendered as akhet ... meaning literally 'place where the great light arises.'

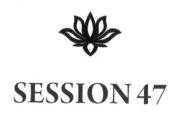

SESSION 47

Angelic Presence

SOURCE: *Gary, one of the things to share with you today are these light beings that are following you around.*

Sondra: Oh, that explains it. I just found a passage in Mary Baker Eddy's book and you're the one I am supposed to read it to. This is in *Science and Health with Key to the Scriptures*, under "Science of Being." Mary said:

> *"Angels are not etherealized human beings evolving animal qualities in their wings. They are celestial visitants flying on spiritual, not material pinions. Angels are pure thoughts from God, winged with truth and love no matter what their individualism may be. Human conjecture confers upon angels its own forms of thought marked with superstitious outlines making them human creatures with suggestive feathers. But this is only fancy. My angels are exalted thoughts; with white fingers, they point upward to a new glorified trust, to higher ideals of life and its joys. Angels are God's representatives. These upward soaring beings never lead towards self, sin or materiality, but guide to divine principle. By giving earnest heed to these spiritual guides, they carry with us and we entertain angels unaware."*

Sondra: So, angels are these light beings?

SOURCE: *Yes, yes. Gary, your mission in this plane, this Earth plane, to reveal them. And the way you reveal them is to allow them presence. Absolutely.*

They're magnificent. They train the highest masters, so they are full of wisdom, righteousness and truth. They direct, guide, uplift, bring people, send people, draw crowds, wake people up, and they cause a ruckus of light and spirituality in gatherings.

Gary, you will be co-creating with these angels. You will have no way not to, because they're now entering your sphere of consciousness. Actually, you are entering their sphere of consciousness. This would be more accurate.

There is an angelic being that adores you above all. And she, although no angel, has a gender; some are just more feminine and some are more masculine. There is a feminine angelic being who refers to her state of being as Eve. So, you can call upon Eve as the light bearer.

Gary: Any specific angelic being to assist me in my greater path of the I Am?

SOURCE: *In angelic form there really isn't a singular one, although you might call upon the archangels. The archangels are big enough to spotlight your path. Archangel Michael is probably your best aligner. Michael is truly the triumphant image of an archangel that you need, the triumphant one.*

Gary: Are there angelic hosts that can assist me in holding a perimeter of light against any entities that would like to subvert our work?

SOURCE: *There's always that. You may indeed call upon the angelic presence that's always wanting to speak with you. You can also enliven the people and to protect the room, the project or the process. That is certainly something that can be in an open prayer to your angelic beings. They are in the light and of the light that you are creating. This is a very good prayer to pray: "Please dismiss any darkness that may be attempting to shut out our light or to shun our light.*[261]

Sondra: Are there any excerpts from Gary's readings that are publishable now?

SOURCE: *Absolutely. If you feel to teach the inner circle some of the concepts such as the Eoma, Blue Flame, human spirit or any other aspect of the readings you find so beautiful. There is no reason you can't create a notebook of excerpts of the master teachings of Gary Springfield. These master teachings channel through Sondra Sneed. But ultimately, this is your Soul which is distilled through language for Sondra. This isn't something that comes from Sondra. She's just the master who knows how to distill it into language.*[262]

---

261   I had been introduced to healing with angels in 1982 when I met and worked with Dorie D'Angelo, the Angel Lady of Carmel. She was a renowned healer, known worldwide. She passed away to the realms of Light two years later at 84 A.Y. (angelic years). She introduced each client to their very own Guardian Angel of Light, and then took them on a healing adventure with their Angel to the special place "their" Angel knew about that was their sacred healing space. This was another confirmation of the majesty and wisdom of the angels co-creating with man/woman. (For those interested I have a couple of free healing tapes from Dorie on my website.)

262   Sondra talked about her work as "Soul readings" and this was a confirmation of her clear ability to touch into another Soul and impart profound information. The paragraph also mentions that I could teach some of these concepts to the inner circle. However, I felt it was so important to get this information out into the world now that I decided to publish the book.

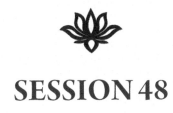

SESSION 48

Torus Knowledge

Gary's comments: Sondra had a session with another client and it was revealed that a sphere (Torus), which is composed of Source mind-energy, creates a point of irritation in order to create knowledge and awareness. The analogy was an oyster with a grain of sand creating a luminescent pearl of beauty from irritation.

Gary: Within my Torus field what is the irritation calling me into higher expression?

SOURCE: *Great question. The first thing that's calling your attention is how far do I exist beyond my body? How far do I enter a dimension from my body? Where is my body relative to me? Who am I that contains a body? So, the Torus is irritating your physical nature. But when you are beyond even your own heart, knowing that you are more than just a heart … you are a mind accelerated in its truth, then your Soul starts to expand beyond your training. You know when you're with people, no matter who they are and how much you care about them, they will always irritate this greater nature of you that wants* *to serve them and expand your knowing.*[263]

Gary: So, I just shine light and love upon them. I suppose it's just like the sun shines light upon me and gives me essence to grow.

SOURCE: *Yes. Shine light upon them, as if it was their surface that's receiving you. What's beyond their surface is their responsibility. Only people who have gone beyond their surface will see you beyond your surface.*

We would add that the Torus is for you and you can only move into it in the right environment. It is not for them that you do it. It is for your discovery of the limit between physical and spirit. This is for your exploration. In the process of you exploring that, people will experience you spiritually, which helps to awaken them.[264]

Gary: Would you say spiritual light is the doorway or portal that is opening for them?

SOURCE: *No. Doorway is a better word. Portal indicates it's a period in time. Portals open and close, they transition with vibration, they have a frequency of connection. That's a portal. Time has a portal.*

A doorway is an illuminant entry point. Doorways are very much guarded at a certain level of awakening. They're guarded by mirrors of self, and anyone who has any dark, seedy sensory systems cannot enter some of these doorways.

---

263   I knew I always looked to serve and expand life. Here I was presented with a deeper understanding that it is really an irritation by the Divine Mind (Torus field) I Am to expand into the higher dimensions. The process of enlightenment is experienced, not by floating away to some magical place, but awakening Higher frequency in the body. These Higher dimensions are within the field of Divine Mind that you expand into for the acknowledgment of Christ within.

264   Healing is not about trying to change things or people. It is about shining a higher vibrational tone upon life (just like the physical sun), which nurtures all things to grow because of its radiance. So too, spiritual illumination shines the light upon those who choose to awaken the light within themselves and grow.

This one in particular requires that the only ones who can walk through this doorway are the ones who are pure.[265]

Sondra: Does the Christ shine on All That Is?

SOURCE: *Yes, yes.*

Sondra: So, this creates the apparition or holographic vision of All That Is?

SOURCE: *Right!*

Sondra: All That Is, is projecting from the Christ … like a projection?

SOURCE: *Right.*

Sondra: All That Is, is just a dream from what the Christ is projecting out to see itself?

SOURCE: *No. It's projecting to make itself, not to see itself. It's projecting to make itself. I am this and I am that … and I am this and I am that. That's what the Christ is making, manifesting.*[266]

---

265   I found this interesting that doorways to spiritual awakening are not guarded by some entity or querulous being, but simply mirror the essence of those who stand at the door. If the reflection is pure and guileless, then the doorway is yours to enter into. The doorway to the revelation of Christ is within one's self.

266   Here is a subtle distinction worth noting: "All That Is, is projecting to make itself, not to see itself." Christ is the mechanism for manifesting unmanifest Source into visible being. God sees what God can be as Christ makes what God IS. The five senses experience the holographic dream as solid reality, but physics tell us that an atom is 99.9999999% space, and the electron is postulated to be a fuzzy mass of thought. The great mystery of creation!

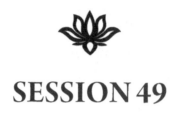

SESSION 49

The Being That Is Ever More

Student #1: Why did we three come together at this time?

SOURCE: *That is a matter of vibration. Vibration draws to itself the signature of its nature. Eventually, all of you who are to be involved in this great awakening, and we mean this in a very different way than most people use the word awakening … we don't mean a whole bunch of people are going to awaken at once. What we mean is, the flower that is blooming is suddenly a representation of what it was always meant to be. There is a blooming that is occurring now, and when it is finally bloomed, the One Hundred will be formed and be speaking on the plane of sound that awakens a huge ripple in a state of the Christ. In that state of the Christ there is a call to, and return call from, the state of God being God. So that's where you're headed. Those who were destined to be a part of this are starting to become closer and closer to each other physically.*[267]

---

267   There were two major aspects of this work with Source. One is to demonstrate and create a pathway for each individual to awaken the Christ condition within. The second is to gather One Hundred illuminated beings and create a unified ignition of the Christ field as a living ripple of "nu-clear" energy for evolving humanity.

Student #2: This is a quote from one of the sessions: "For the human race this could result in a majority of the human race being wiped out."

SOURCE: *The way to see it is, what is the path of human existence? Human existence is on a path to non-existence as it wipes out all of the resources that are necessary to sustain a human existence. Then it is on a path of extinction.*

Student #2: I hear behind this or feel there is some notion that human evolution could be lost.

SOURCE: *Well, you make it sound as if that is a conscious effort by some larger entity, is that what?*

Student #2: No, I feel as though what is taking place more accurately is the Earth and humanity has been hijacked by corporate greed and possibly alien influences, and what would be appropriate would be to clear the infestation and provide an opportunity for positive next steps.

SOURCE: *Well, you're correct in assuming there are ways of changing the consciousness of the human world, where they are not so trained to create in the course of destruction. However, the time it would take to retrain humans en masse will be too late before the resources necessary to sustain a human existence would survive.*

Student #2: Unless there is technology introduced to the equation.

SOURCE: *You cannot technologically replace forests, wildlife, streams, rivers and the natural course of evolution that created the planet. There is no technology that would make that possible.*

Student #2: Consciousness can terraform the planet in a matter of a blink of an eye actually, the entire thing.

SOURCE: *Well, in the grand scheme of things, this 26,000-year cycle is the blink of an eye. It takes thousands of years to rebuild forests in a way that they are producing highly diverse ecosystems.*

When the Earth is less than 65% forest, there is a mechanism in the Earth that says time to wipe out whatever is on the surface of the planet and engage in the next phase of evolution. Evolution is an evolving system that is recorded in the history of the planet. And it is recorded in the way the planet is in orbit, how it is on its axis. So, what adjusts the axis of a planet that is moving in its stages of evolution are fully and completely in alignment with how the systems are working together. When a planet is completely off balance to the point where it cannot regrow itself, then the turning and the churning of the planet takes place. And the change of the axis is based on mechanisms with intricate structures like a clock.

Student #1: Okay, so what's the big deal about surviving? From my understanding of studying esoteric literature, life and death is not really that much of a difference from that higher viewpoint. So why is it such a big deal?

SOURCE: *Well, this is the part that humans get hung up on. Humans think they are the only ones on this planet that are in need of the planet, so they can just wipe it out and if they get wiped out in the process, who cares? But that's not the case. There are many worlds that depend on the existence of this planet and all of the resources that are on this planet. There are worlds upon worlds upon worlds that require this remains a productive planet. It is all God, and it is a process of God that replicates itself based on its own creative presentation. So, as it presents itself in the way that it is, it notices itself in the pureness of its greatness. But if all it sees of itself is its own destruction, it becomes a confluence of destruction until it is no more, and that is a spread of the nothingness.*[268]

---

268   It sounds rather harsh when Source is talking about an extinction event, but human ignorance and greed have raped the planet. The dynamic ecological mechanisms of Earth will create a new evolution with or without humanity. That is why the stated purpose of this work is to implement a new understanding of the creative process through the Christing system. This will allow humanity to live in Oneness with Nature/Spirit and co-create a new human/divine evolution on Earth.

Gary: (There was a long pause where we had no more questions and so a story was offered.)

SOURCE: *We could tell a story if you wanted to hear a story.*

Student #1: I would love a story.

SOURCE: *Once upon a time there was a system that had no order to it. And this system started to question its existence. It started to wonder if there was order, and what kind of order would this order be. So, it started to feel its edges and as it attempted to know where its edges were, it saw it had no edges at all; it just went on and on and on. It tried to find some sense of the final part in order for it to fold over to make itself its first fold in an order of order.*

Then it saw that it could make more of itself just by finding what it thought was its edge and it expanded. When it suddenly saw it was expanding as it reached, it reached from all sides of itself, and it reached further into what it could not see, what it could not experience in its sense of itself. It just knew it was reaching and reaching and reaching. One day, when it was tired of reaching and reaching and wanted to come back to itself, it wanted to feel its center again; it was tired of the outer reaches, the reaches that went on forever to nowhere, to no thing, even though it was creating something.

But it still didn't feel like home anymore, so it came back and started its journey back to its center. As it made its way back to its center, it realized it never left its center at all. It had always been there; even in its furthest reaches it had always been right there in its center.

So, it decided to find a way to be both in its center and in its outer reaches too. How could it know itself and its greatest part of itself and be in the place that is warm and comfortable, how could it be comfortable too? So, it asked itself this question, "How can I know me that is the center of me and also be the greatest of me?" This me, that it asked of itself, said back to itself, "Just make a new me and I'll show you in the new me what is the greater of me and you just practice being that me." So, the being that had no order, that didn't know how far it could go, and didn't know its center at all, started to formulate something of what it thought it was, and made another one. And when it did, it saw how magnificent it was, it saw the mirror of itself and it said, "Is that me ... that's me?" And it said back to itself, "It's me, it's me!" And in the mirror of itself that it saw, it saw its edges reach toward itself.

So, it made a new me, of the one that it always was, in the center of itself, a new one that it is now. The new one that is the old one, and the new one together, even bigger than the first one.

As it began this process of mirroring itself over and over, finding out what this me is, this greater and greater of me that it became, it saw that it could make other 'me' that were the exact opposite of this me, and in that opposite, it began to build for the first time a system of order; the me not-me system of order. It was the on and the off, the in and the out, the up and the down. It began to fall in love with this amazing process of me not-me, me not-me, me not-me and everything it made in diversity of this thing, it explored in conversation of what it could be. And it offered itself suggestions, and in those suggestions there were more suggestions, and each suggestion made a new suggestion, and each suggestion that made a new suggestion was a brand-new picture of me. And in this beautiful suggestion there was a making of the order of new. And newness became the awareness of the All ... as it reached back to itself every time it called to the outer and it brought to the inner. Each call to the outer was a new inner and each new inner was a suggestion for what it oozed out of itself to be. In the final days, when it said, "I am bored," suddenly a new eruption would happen, and that eruption would delight it and it would crawl out of its shell, out of its center, and that center would die as it made a new shell.

Each time it made a new shell, because it was bored, it realized it created a nothing from its boredom; it died when it was bored. So, it said, "I need a new system; this system must delight me always, it must always make me more me."

So, it created color and created joy, and it found that in joy ... as it followed joy, it knew itself newly. The more that it knew itself newly, the more beautiful and spectacular it became to itself and it never again denied itself joy in being what it is.

This is each one of you, each one of you is a joy in pursuit to find the thing that is making joy, and every time you find this thing that is making joy within you, you live and you keep living forever more, for the fear of dying is greater than the effort of finding joy.[269]

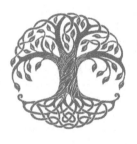

---

269   I included this beautiful and magical story of Source creating and recreating itself to reaffirm for you and me that We are Source, re-creating life and expanding the universe. You are One with God.

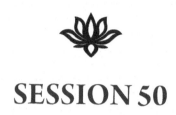

SESSION 50

Multidimensional Awareness

Gary: My body is going through quite a bit of discomfort because of the new alignments in meditation. I think I'm living more outside the physical form and the body doesn't appreciate it.

SOURCE: *Your field is triggering pain in the body. It's not the body itself, it's the field. The body is an inoperable field of energy with regard to the spiritual field of energy.*

The multi-dimensional meditation you are doing is the want of you to go beyond the body. The body doesn't want you to exit it. The body (as you recognized) wants you in it; otherwise, it feels as if it has no meaning, and doesn't have a purpose. If you can walk around without a body, then why do you need a body? And the body starts to freak out. It is experiencing pain in the process of being left behind, essentially in the parameter of death. There is a window where it lives and dies, a window of its perception. In the living and dying perception, the body is experiencing pain to forewarn itself; if it doesn't reconnect it's going to die. So, to desensitize that means reaching further than that in order to incorporate the feeling of being just outside the body.

This is very different than people who astral travel. It's not the same thing. You are expanding the Soul's reach. People who travel astrally aren't incorporating the body at all. They're moving from thought wave to thought wave. Their Soul is on a journey in an astral plane.

You are having a Soul expansion experience. In that Soul expansion you are doing what a Soul is capable of doing without a body, when the Soul is identified as a separate entity from the body. Most people cannot separate those two things. Even if someone astral travels, they immediately, upon waking, return to the systems of the body. You aren't doing that, that's not the nature of the work. You are not returning to the systems of the body, you are governing the systems of the body … but the body is not your parameter of existence.

For someone who astral travels at night in their out-of-body experiences, they're leaving the body on a course of thought train movement. You're in spirit train movement.

As you walk across the floor outside of your body, the only way you know you're walking (as opposed to flying) *is selective-sensory sensation. You're selecting the bottom of your feet to feel. If you select the top of your head, you might feel the texture of the ceiling because you've chosen to experience you from the top of your head. Then you move to your feet and feel the floor. You suddenly realize how tall you are. Your head is hitting the ceiling and your feet are hitting the floor. That's the objective.*

The sensory identifier needs to move around the desensitized pain receptors and become more reaching. The receptors need to reach further into and beyond the connection to the body. The body is the mind processing the feel of texture. The body is identifying the difference between textures. It's noticing where (in the condition that you are in) the sensation is when you are walking across the floor. It's identifying the three-dimensional feedback of where you are.[270]

Sondra: That's interesting. It seems counter-intuitive to what many people think they're doing when they're out-of-body traveling. They think they're on a spiritual train.

SOURCE: *Well, that's because there's no distinction between Soul and Spirit. There is a huge distinction between Soul and Spirit. Most people do not make that distinction. They think the journey of their soul is a spiritual journey, but it's a thought journey. They travel into their imagination and the imagination can go into worlds that exist, but they exist on an imaginary plane. It's not that they don't exist in another dimension, it's just that they can only be visited through the imaginary plane because the imagination is the construct of that existence. It is a world that was imagined, built and then contains the imagination of what it was built into. Therefore, anyone who visits in a condition of the travel is doing so in and through imagination. Gary's spring field is a completely different level of striation. The dimension on which Gary is interacting has to be somewhere in the fourth and fifth dimension. He's entering a fourth and fifth dimensional shift for his own experience of the interaction. The experience is what gives him a feeling of my foot is on the floor, my head is on the ceiling.*

---

270   One of the important parts of this work was to achieve an existence of living outside the body as well as "having" a body. Human beings have become singularly focused on the body and have lost touch with the divine quality that exists eternally, that lives in spirit. However, it did cause a fair amount of pain as I was learning how to be outside the body.

Sondra: I have a question, is the spring field the Torus?

SOURCE: *No. The Torus is created from the Spring Field. It's springing and the condition of this is the everlasting life. We'll just call it that, the everlasting life, ever giving, ever building, and ever creating. This ever condition is forever and ever and ever. It is what is springing. The field from that spring, then, is everything that is made in the process of the everlasting, and a Torus is certainly a condition of that spring. It's not the only one; it's just one condition of it. It's what gives a sphere its magnetic change. How it changes and alters in its magnetic field is the torrent, the Torus current.*[271] (Spring field in Source terms is not referring specifically to Gary's last name, but to the field of reality that springs from the open doorway into the void, which the Christ illuminates.)

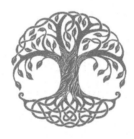

---

271 The magnetic stroke of the Torus field, in its flowing movement, is similar to the magnetic lines of force that surround Earth and extend far out into space. In the human Torus, there is a constant springing forth of life that flows up to the top of the Torus field, then all around and back up through the body again. The "spring field" arises forth from the inner dimensions within the heart chakra; the heart is often referred to as the engine of God. The breath and the magnetic stroke of the Torus (Divine mind) generate life.

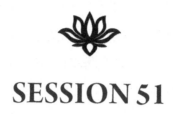

SESSION 51

Christe Field Eminence

Sondra: Gary, based on what I've experienced in your readings and what you propel in the silence of meditation, I am perfectly comfortable saying that Christ is not Jesus. "Jesus was illuminated by the Christ" is now projected from the Christ and that light is Chrism, C H R I S M, like prism, like Christ-prism, light and water.

Gary: That is a beautiful revelation. I've also come to the knowing as a result of these sessions and my own experience that the void mastered the Christ in order to make itself; i.e., to see itself. The Christ is the doorway back into Source creation. Christ is the way. Christ is the only way. Jesus, Mary or Gary can be the way, but the way is really the Self, which is through the Christ-prism within.

Sondra: And it's prismatic, prism-matic.

Gary: That's good. In the very first Source dialogue we did five years ago, it was said (and I will paraphrase), "Christ consciousness does have a way of sustaining itself in individuation, provided there is a room that is given a sanctimonious prism."

SOURCE: *It is the prism from which all light reveals the interior state. All light reveals the interior state through the prismatic event, known geometrically as* *the star tetrahedron. It's actually the refractions of light interacting that are the event. These star tetrahedrons multiply on each other within their origin, reflect from their origin, and express out of some density impossible to describe in words.*[272]

Gary: How can my inner alignment to the Christ and the work I am to do be increased?

SOURCE: *You can be more of a Soul without a body among those who know you. Practice appearing in their dreams, in their room, their car or in their periphery. Start to create a witness to your appearance. Keep a journal of what your experience is of that, and consistently do it so that you can watch changes in these experiences. Perhaps during the first month of these Soul appearances (without a body) you struggle with certain aspects/details, or you struggle to know if it's working. What are the parts that are easy? What are the parts that seem hard? In the next month you can identify what is the experience of being in their presence? Do they personally affect the process or were they personally affected?*

In your mind's eye you create the feeling of their presence. From this feeling of their presence, you become present to where they are. This process should give you a picture of what you think they're doing. It may not always be obvious, but

---

272   I thought it was astounding that information from our very first dialogue, (7 years ago) was now being alluded to and edified. The focusing of consciousness hones and refines light/love into a living jewel. This is the mystical marriage that creates the prismatic form of the multi-faceted star tetrahedron. From this prismatic jewel there is an emanation, an energetic wave … this is the Christ field that creates life. The interior state mentioned in the paragraph above is the void, which the Christ illuminates. The corresponding light refractions (through the prismatic jewel) creates holographic life. The Eoma precipitates that image into form and the five senses interpret this as physical reality.

remember to take notes.[273]

Gary: In one of our sessions the Egyptian pyramids were referenced in their relationship to the Christ consciousness.

SOURCE: *Yes, we don't call it Christ consciousness. That's a palatable term that allows non-Christians to Christianize their spirituality. Our word is a Christ field, much the way in a nuclear explosion there's a field that emanates from the epicenter. It's not a consciousness (that field) because it's not a singular state of mind. It's a singular being that reproduces multiplicity of being. It expresses being, and in the expression of being that is the Christ, individuals who reflect back inwardly to their origin of the Christ (in the Christ) become a Christed nature or become anointed in the Christ. They achieve Christos; they illuminate from within to equalize the light from within to the without, and from the without to the within. They emanate, so the Christ field is within an individual emanation. This emanation replicates the state of God-being which unifies the Higher Self with the material self. The illuminated Self represents a state of God's nature in its individual way and true way. The Origin is reflecting back to itself (you) … and returning Itself (God) … to that which is looking upon it (you). You are God. And that which is looking upon it has a Christ condition. That is not a consciousness.*

Consciousness is a collection of processes that returns memory and thought. Consciousness collects, organizes and delivers mind. It contains the individual and the collective of all individuals within. Consciousness is to thought the

---

273   The eternal Soul appropriates a body each lifetime in order to gain experiential wisdom. Over time, the realization dawns that you can learn how to live beyond the body in consciousness while you are embodied. A challenging task because the body is in survival-fear, and sometimes reacts with pain as you rise into these higher dimensions. With each meditation you look for a new way to soothe and love the body as you move into each new adjustment. It was recommended that I imagine, feel and breathe more spirit/space between all the molecules of the body, and this assisted me.

way mist is to water. Consciousness is vapor of thought, electrical, and can be triggered. It can create a thunderstorm of process of mind. Christ field raptures itself of itself and doesn't need the consciousness of an individual to be itself. It doesn't need the consciousness of the whole to be itself, because it constantly recreates without thought. The Christ can exist without thought and consciousness cannot. Consciousness is interpreting itself all the time.

What am I? I Am.

Where am I? I am here.

What is here? Here is now.

What is now? Now is here.

Who is here? I am here.

Christ field takes those thoughts and makes from them; makes anything those thoughts think. Thoughts are a command to the Christ. Christ produces what those thoughts think, and with each "I am" that thought is thinking, the Christ dictates what it is by what it mirrors in the IT... that is asking what IT is.

That is a clarification when considering what you are, that is Illuminating, as the Christ becomes apparent within you ... as you light up in pure silence.[274]

Gary: Is this why it is being spoken more and more that I need to be in silence? Because the Christ is not a thought or thinking, it's just pure being in the unity of God expressing?

---

274   A beautiful description of the Christ field and how it differs from old, outdated perceptions and religious connotations. Many of the preceding dialogues find their culmination in this profound declaration; Christ is not an individual, it is a nu-clear field of energy ... it is the very cornerstone of Original creation. In its individual way it can represent God on Earth through you and I when we achieve Christos. The creative field of the Christ system is the creation of the universe, reflecting into form unmanifest God within the void ... to make what God can be.

SOURCE: *Right, right. The unity of God expressing is a mechanism of creation. Creation is the attempt to organize in consciousness. All that is thought and dreamed makes some version of these thoughts and dreams in order to see what has been thought and dreamed.*

The quiet, silent mind hangs in the Christ. It just hangs there. It's not processing thought in order to force the Christ to create. It's in the zero point. It's hovering in the zero point. From this zero point then, if you control your thoughts in a creative way where you create and it creates you, the Christ listens to these thoughts in order to interpret into being what you are thinking.

Thought dictates to the Christ what to make and there is nothing until there is silence; then you're at zero. You can take a bad situation and you create a no-thought state, which completely devours the bad situation into nothingness. It no longer exists until you remember it in that way as a bad situation. You can recreate the situation from that zero point into any situation you choose.

Sondra: So that means it would create negative things from negative thought.

SOURCE: *Of course, it means that. It has no judgment or opinion. Doesn't see it as negative or positive. It just sees it as is. So you say … it shall be, that's all the Christ sees. So you say … it shall be, amen, it is so.*

The Christ overtakes the thought mind potential of a person who is ailing and changes the dynamic of their thought by bringing it energetically to zero point. This redirects the thought process after zero from trauma to tremendous.[275]

---

275   Zero-point is a state of no thought and is pure crystalline consciousness. In this pure silence the Christ can dissolve the "thought/light form" that has an appearance of reality, and then re-image-in the wholeness and perfection of Source/God to create healing. In its highest expression the Christ field can effortlessly manifest loaves and fishes … all possibilities within the mind of God become manifest through the Christ system.

SESSION 52

Eoma Love Intelligence

SOURCE: *We are talking about Golden Light emanating from the Christ. The edges of the Christ are the crystalline foundation of all manifestation that comes out of matter. Matter manifests from the Christ through this crystalline structure that multiplies in every prismatic direction. Through every direction of the prism, it creates a new direction, and every new direction multiplies, multiplies, multiplies. Every new direction of a "what's next, where do I go … what's next, where do I go," is a new creation, a manifestation of thought. Where thought leads. "Where do I go?"*

Thought leads (where do I go) in a prismatic manner, so that it moves in the direction of its creation. That what It is creating is that what It is, and It is identifying that creation at the same time It is being that creation … and It is unifying from a singular creation. It then becomes one with the unity of what is making It. It no longer needs a reflection of itself … the "what" It is. It is looking at itself directly from its interior origin. This interior origin can redirect the entirety of an experience when the experience goes from origin to place of being in a single light stroke. As strokes happen in the body, they happen for the benefit of the body just as readily as they happen for the non-benefit of the body. The light stroke must be taken in a channeled way through to the origin and the healed whole self … at the same time that it is a bi-directional expression of its true state. As soon as it does this it heals itself in its understanding and redirects an orientation when the thought looks back at itself from its physical state. Healing within the Christed beam is a representation of an original thought. The whole thought, not just whisper or part. When the whole thought is spoken to the body and the whole thought of the body is remembered in its whole way, it is identifying itself as a Christ.[276]

Gary: When we are hanging in void, in the zero point, it's a no-thought state. Do I focus the light of the mind upon an image/feeling?

SOURCE: *Absolutely. Focus the mind upon an image/feeling. That is step one, and each new step, new step arrives at the next step. It's the power of the imagination to make what is real view-able ... through the true real in each moment.*

Gary: The *true real* is hovering in the void as the fullness of Source oneness?

SOURCE: *Yes.*

Gary: Once we reach zero point, we are hovering in the void, and there is a density all around. When we have an image/feeling, it would manifest?

SOURCE: *Yes.*

---

276   The Christ mechanism is creation. When one identifies with this system and rests within this creative principle, one creates from inside out ... and views each new creation as they expand into it; i.e., "Where do I go, what's next?" Imagine you are the breath that is blowing a bubble. As you breathe more into the bubble (you are inside the bubble) it expands and from that interior perspective you are watching the creative expansion. You are not sitting on the outer surface looking at things around you as a reflection, you are the interior creator. When you identify with this creative principle, you are looking at yourself as Source/God creating healing and renewal from the healed whole self, as well as expanding life around you in eternal glory. In a single "light stroke" of perception you can identify your Divine Origin, heal trauma in the body or psyche, illuminating evermore the individual Christ I Am.

Gary: Within the Christed system as you identify the image/feeling within the void is it the Eoma arising forth simultaneously from out of the void that makes the image/feeling coordinate within time-space?

SOURCE: *No. The Eoma is dwelling in a multi-dimensional plane experience, absolutely. But this isn't a concerted state of the Christ. The Christ and the Eoma interact in that the Eoma is sent where life must be. The Eoma is sent were life must be. Not all of the Christ is pure light; sometimes it's crescent. Pure light systems without crescent are like lightning running across the sky, it is a reaction.*

There is a light that is a reaction and then there is a light that is a living. In the light that is living there lives the Eoma. That answers the question regarding how the Eoma and Christ field unite. They are uniting in the living. All that is alive is dwelling within this layer that is also known as love.[277]

Sondra: The Eoma and love are united?

SOURCE: *No. Eoma is in love with love. Eoma never separates from love, it refuses to separate from love. It could if it wanted; it could be an ooze outside of love, but it chooses always to love. The Eoma is a foundation of pure. It holds pure in space. It makes space, gives space, dwells within the space, holds space. Eoma is critical to Gary's work because it is space and it holds him. Eoma holds him, gives him love, shows him love and cares for him. It's in every essence. Eoma is powerful because it works very hard to protect its own.*

---

277   The Eoma is ubiquitous throughout time/space but in a "dimension" that is unseen with the physical senses. The prismatic Christ field creates a reflection of light out of the void which calls the Eoma into precipitation around the holographic image and coalesces into form. The Eoma is the very essence of love and it "so loves" what light reflects, that it gathers around these light images. Christ is the mechanism and the Eoma is the substance.

Gary: What's the relationship between the breath and the Eoma?

SOURCE: *The Eoma is all that is alive. Breath is breathing life. If you breathe from the Eomic field you're calling in that layer of love-life that creates. It creates an environment in the body to receive a healing or it creates in the body the ability to heal from working out. It is a perpetuating machine of living life. Even life that is dying it is still living in a new direction from the Eomic field.*[278]

Gary: What is the "word" spoken of in the Bible?

SOURCE: *Consciousness. In the beginning was consciousness and the consciousness was with God. Consciousness then became aware of itself in the void. That awareness is the Christ. Consciousness seeing itself became self-aware and thus created the light of the Christ … it fell in love with itself. It's always falling in love with itself. God sees what God can be, and it is love. Creation is love.*[279]

---

278   It is important to remember that even though the Eoma is the essence of love, it can only reflect that which you feel or think it to be. If you unconsciously breathe negative thoughts and feelings into the ubiquitous Eoma, it disrupts the systems of the body rather than heals. Imagine wholeness, health, love and joy, and so it shall be!

279   New Testament, John 1: In the beginning was the Word, and the Word was with God, and the Word was God. 2 He was with God in the beginning. 3 Through him all things were made; without him nothing was made that has been made. 4 In him was life, and that life was the light of all mankind. 5 The light shines in the darkness, and the darkness has not overcome it.

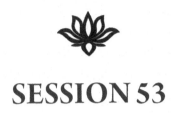

SESSION 53

The Foundation of The Christ

Gary: I often feel illuminated and dynamic but then there are periods of discomfort and burning in the body that is quite uncomfortable at times.

Sondra: What happens to Gary when this is going on?

SOURCE: *Well, you are a star feature. The condition of the stars in certain star alignments will disassemble your ground. You are ungrounded which leads to all kinds of damage in the process.*

The only time you can go into a grounded state is when the stars are aligned for you, which is when your spirit is strong. It's weakened when you enter fortified fields of electromagnetic churn that comes from your potent meditations. It exhausts your spirit in a good way. It expands your spirit to beyond your body.

In the exhaustion you struggle to ground because you're floating. You're a floating orb from these meditations and there's no reason to ground as a floating orb, unless you're still a body. When you're still a body, the electromagnetic field attacks the body if the body is not grounded.

When we say star feature, we mean the stellar, celestial body that is a giant orb of light full of fantastic, innumerable, creative potential. Everything comes out of the celestial body known as the sun, in the center of a solar system. That sun is itself a creation for creation … an orb of creation for creation. It's God's happy place. In God's happy place God expands what God is from that happy place and waits for <u>environmental perfection</u> to express God's Self in the Christed state.

As God expresses God's Self in the Christed state, all manner of potential comes from this. All the beautiful beings come out of this process of God expressing God's Self being in the nature of God's way. A Christed etheric mechanism is utilized by a Christ Child to be one with the Father. This represents a foundation, (not a male parent but foundation) and is the foundation of that which is becoming.

In the foundation of that which is becoming, there is a new creation that is birthing the foundation of the Mother, in order that the Father can create from God's Self. The Mother was made by the Father as a perfection of that which was the foundation. I am perfect, I make what is perfect, I need that which is making to be perfect. I need that which is making in order to <u>per-fect</u>, and that which is making is that which is birthing. The foundation of Father/Mother is holding inside of "itself" to then draw from "itself "some version of "itself." Mother nature is the constant birthing of nature that is experienced on a planet, which begins in the core of creation, and in the core of that creation is a sun. The sun that is in the heavens is also in the liquid core of the planet because the planet is experiencing a birthing of the origin.

The Christ Child is the one born under the star, and that star is a celestial event, just as the Christ which comes from the Father is a celestial event.

The Mother is the mother of invention, a Mother nature. It's not a Mother in the way of a parent any more than God the Father is the father or a male parent. It is foundation, and then it is re-creation from the foundation that is Mother.[280]

Sondra: Creation is a re-creation?

SOURCE: *Yes, from the Foundation, from the Origin.*

Sondra: And a Christ Child is here to do what?

SOURCE: *Train the event. Train the event.*

Sondra: The event of Revelation?

SOURCE: *Correct. Life forever and ever more in revelation. Life ever more is from the one who is aware that they create what they experience. That they experience what they create. The one that is experiencing a creation from self-awareness is in full control of their experience. This is a profound moment for the Soul; one is the inventor of one's own experience.*

The Christ is not a consciousness, it's the mechanism of creation. A consciousness is an organized state of individuality, individual. The Christ is not consciousness, it is a manifesting mechanism, the Creator itself. It is the creator.

---

280   In meditation it often feels that sunlight is emanating from me, and the process of ushering my body into the higher vibrational tones to accommodate this energy is my daily practice. Also, the description of how the Origin re-creates itself as a sun within a solar system and then creates more life from that stellar origin is beautiful … God's happy place. The physical sun is a Christ mechanism on a cosmic level. All planets are birthed from a sun, and within the molten core of Earth is a Christ mechanism, revealing Its identity in the evolution of all life on the planet; i.e., Mother nature. A man/woman can be a Christ sun on a human level … replicating God's light on Earth. This Self-revelation is an important component of the Earth's Christing. Enlightened humans will become the symbolic neurons of memory and higher intelligence that will co-create with Gaia/Earth the Heaven on Earth experience.

The Christ is the way all is created. When an individual becomes self-aware enough to incorporate the Christ in one's self-identity, one is in control of all one creates. The Christ interacts with consciousness, is very much a part of consciousness, but is not in and of itself a consciousness. In fact, it cannot ever become conscious of itself or it would implode. The Christ is a projection from itself. If it ever looked back at itself, it would turn back into zero point.[281]

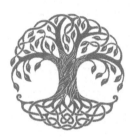

---

281   The analogy of the breath blowing a bubble is also relevant here. If you were the eternal breath and expanding your bubble of creation (as an individualized Christ), then stopped in order to look at "who is blowing this bubble", the cessation of breath would collapse the bubble. That is zero point ... no thought, no being ... the void once again. The Christ field is able to hover at the doorway to the void and illuminate thought/image, in order to reflect it into a dimensional world to make what God can be. The Christ is the Light/Lens of creation; i.e., the projection of Source into dimensional reality. I AM ... is the ever expanding breath (bubble) of creation.

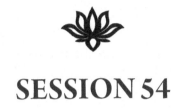

SESSION 54

Earth Changes

Sondra: What is the current state of humanity's relationship with Earth?

SOURCE: *The current relationship with man and with Earth cannot coincide. The Earth cannot receive what man is. Until man loves the Earth as himself, the Earth rejects all that does not love it back. It will do whatever it can to shake man off of it. Earth is a fragile nature, and it can easily remove that which abuses it. But not until man has already destroyed the fragile natures.*

The human vessel is a misrepresentation of man because the human vessel is so far different from the man that was made in the image of God.

Sondra: Are there other vessel humanoid creatures that are also man?

SOURCE: *Yes.*

Sondra: Do they exist in alien form?

SOURCE: *No. They are on other Earths. They are a process of an Earthen nature. Things that are not of an Earth are un-terrestrial.*

Gary: Are the individuals within the Galactic Federation a replica of the human form?

SOURCE: *The Galactic Federation are representatives of Peace among regents.*

(*Sondra looks up Regency from the dictionary*: Is the office of, or period of government by a regent. A regent is a person appointed to administer a country, administering because the monarch is a minor or is absent or is incapacitated.)

Sondra: So, God, are you the monarch or is Jesus?

SOURCE: *No. The human world has lost its king. The human world has no principles, it has no government. It has territories, and it has allies. But it is, as a whole, ungoverned. War must be outlawed because man cannot be allowed in space until war is outlawed, until violence and destruction is mitigated. You can't go into space a warring nation or warring people.*

There is a government in space and that government is governed by principles. Those principles are identified as freedom, peace, will to know, the expansion of knowledge, the expansion of discovery and to Be and let Be. There are some Intergalactic provinces that are not so clear on those things. The Christ field ensures that these principles of Life and Liberty are upheld.

Sondra: God loses interest?

SOURCE: Yes.

Sondra: I get the sense there are some creatures in which God has lost interest.

SOURCE: *Yes, in full wretchedness. It is certain that man is on the way to walking outside of God, giving God no reason to remain. God has no interest in God's creations living one over the other. But without some principle of living among, God cannot walk among. It's just that God would lose interest in man altogether if there was no way to govern God within man.*

Much energy, effort, and drive has been spent on mortal man's survival that if mortal man is not concerned with his own survival, what more can be done, but to allow mankind to experience the consequences and start anew.

You are among the ambassadors of man's last chance to experience spiritual regeneration. This must take place if there is to be any hope for the current trajectory of humanity.

Sondra: There are others, though, they have missions too?

SOURCE: *Yes, but what is that to you?*

Sondra: We can't carry it all. All by ourselves. Can we?

SOURCE: *You give little credence to the work that lives on after you. People think that Jesus's work was some giant thing in the time he lived, and it wasn't. It was small, communal, very enclosed. It was only after his death that it became slowly, over time, over century after century of retelling the story, retelling the story, that it became some significant, widespread following. It just wasn't back then.*

The Apostles finally had to sit down and tell his story in order that it would not die with them. It was on the verge of dying with them as they got old. And those stories the Apostles told were written down and passed around, and it grew. But long after the death of Jesus and long after the death of the Apostles and Mary.

Gary: Question. Is there more we can do to uphold our particular missions?

SOURCE: *We would like to have a better question. Is there more we can do to uphold our missions is too projective. It projects into some future, something you should do you aren't doing. So, the question would probably be better, when will the momentum of our mission be realized? And we would say, so long as you continue to plug away in the way that you are doing it, you will come to a merging of resources that wraps it all up, gives it all a nice tight bond.*

It's with that tight bond that the future is imminent as to what the purpose of this work is. For now, you both grope in the dark for what is the reasoning behind the little things you're doing. Sondra suffers tremendously knowing how much there has to be done and having only a tiny amount of energy to complete each day some small portion of what a day is filling for her. Gary is always rather worried and wondering, am I doing enough? Am I doing enough? Is this going to be enough? Is there more I should be doing? These are the conditions of every minister who sees the end could be coming. Who knows that humans are in trouble.

In this way, it has been this way for centuries, centuries upon centuries because man has lost his grip on the Earth before. And it is inevitable that it will happen again. This is the reason you are in these missions, though, to touch as many Souls as possible who will be ready for the next phase of human evolution. They become part of the new evolution that populates the Earth after this evolution of mortal man is complete.

Your only true job before you pass is to establish as many relationships as possible who are among the Souls to evolve.

Gary: So to recap: The energizing of the spirit of man, in conjunction with the Christing that is taking place, is the new program, and simply educating those we can.

SOURCE: *Yes. Yes. Those who participate in that new program are among the new humans, and are the hope of humanity because without them God loses interest. God has lost interest in the past in man. It wasn't until man rediscovered God that God rediscovered man. When God lost interest in man was when man was only interested in himself. This is a time of civilization long gone, long gone. No remnant of that time of civilization still exists. Not even an archaeological remnant that has been discovered, anyway, that exists. This was when the Earth was truly magnificent in so many animal forms. Man became an intellectual superior, and through that superiority thought himself superior.*

Sondra: Atlantis?

SOURCE: *Yes, you are on it. You are aware now to the condition that man is heading toward in which man is in trouble. A planet filled with creatures so self-absorbed, having turned away from the very life-force that created and sustains them (and Earth) to the point of imminent human extinction.*

In the distant past, Atlantis was at the epicenter of an earthquake that created a tsunami. It was wiped out in a tsunami. It was time for the planet to begin to evolve.[282]

We can only warn those who are in states of mindfulness as the restructuring occurs. They will feel it before they see it. They will start to naturally move to areas of safety. They will naturally move to places that are not in the destructive patterns.[283]

---

282 Plato described the story of Atlantis as a civilization that existed about 9,000 years before his own time, and this legend had been passed down by poets, priests, and shamans. The founders of Atlantis, he said, were half god and half human. They created a utopian civilization and became a great naval power.

283 The travail before humanity can still be mitigated if and when enough individuals realize the importance of critical change and act decisively, (and in consort) with governments worldwide. As planetary systems continue to deteriorate each individual must become more attuned to the intuitive voice of wisdom that speaks thought the heart and take the necessary steps one is directed to take. Personal ambition must turn to Global recognition.

🪷 🪷 🪷

Gary's Closing Statement

My opening statement in the introduction summarizes my deep and clear feelings: "I have no fear or worry about the future. I know that Higher intelligence is always co-creating more possibilities with humanity and each individual … if they are open. If people don't hear, then pain and suffering from self-inflicted sabotage becomes their unconscious choice. Earth is an evolving "Being." Nature is always transforming the planet into a new and more exquisite environment.

Have no fear, live in joy, purpose your life from your heart and trust in the divine to lead you into righteousness and welfare (well-fare) during this great transition. Allow yourself to rest in the clear knowing that the transformation into spiritual peace, prosperity and joy is yours to have … if you are clearly listening to your inner guidance … not the ignorance and cacophony of the world. This book will help you clearly understand how your conscious, and more often, unconscious, choices create your reality.

This book is a condensed version taken from the original information. It illuminates the process for accelerated instruction into the embodiment of the Christ condition. It felt important and even critical to share this teaching with humanity as this time.

I still cherish the desire to further codify the process into a precise step-by-step manual, omitting the dialogue, and provide a concise, small handbook for the aspirant. The impact and awakening from this process in my life has been far beyond my expectations, and I wish this enlightened experience for you!

The old adage, "many are called but few are chosen," simply means you must choose yourself to rise to the mountaintop of the Higher Being you are.

❦ ❦ ❦

The Awakening

Spirituality fell into my lap when I was a sophomore in college. A friend gave me a book about the renowned prophet and psychic Edgar Cayce. When I read it, I realized "they" had lied to me … there was another reality besides the life of pain and struggle most people experienced. Shortly thereafter, I was in the local bookstore and three leather-bound books I could not have reached on a top shelf jumped out onto the floor. *Life and Teachings of the Masters of the Far East* was the title. When I took them home and read them, I knew this was Truth. I knew then my life would be dedicated to finding those who knew this truth and lived it.

I began reading every book on spirituality, religion and esoteric lore I could find. Over the following years I filled my mind to the brim with wisdom, but still did not live it in my life. I was a good person, but did not love or honor myself from the deep childhood wounds I carried. Confused and disillusioned by the inconsistency of what I knew and what I lived, I sold my possessions and moved to Carmel, California to find some answers. It was clearly my Soul destiny because I met Dorie D'Angelo, the "Angel Lady of Carmel." She was 82 years old, and a saint who lived, walked and talked love and grace. She took me under her wing and showed me how the power of love can heal any condition, reawaken childlike magic, and open the door to the divine and sacred Soul within.

The discipline of meditation and my devout spiritual practice quickly opened doorway after doorway into the realms of spirit, and before long I was teaching others how to create their sacred relationship with the Soul. Some people would call this divine Self the Christ Consciousness, others the Buddha Nature, and the Jewish tradition would name it the Shekinah Light, but it is all the same Divine and Sacred-Self from Source Oneness.

I opened a healing center in Sedona, Arizona, in 2003 and facilitated workshops and healing retreats. The center housed 20 individuals, which allowed us to be together in a sacred space, meditating and enlivening the divine Soul within. There were two main aspects to the teaching. First and foremost was the meditation. Students were taught how to image/feel the Golden Light of the Soul flowing in and through the body. The innate perfection within the Soul *is* the Divine Self, and that realization in the physical body opens the door to the Christ system. The second part was emotional clearing. Relationship issues, addictions, weight problems and most diseases have their roots in emotional trauma; it is often unconscious. I trained myself to see/feel the aura in order to discern the colors, emotions, past life trauma, and spiritual evolution of an individual. I taught students how to see/feel emotional blockages within themselves, and then I could validate their perceptions or direct them deeper into their own healing.

The numerous workshops I facilitated, along with hundreds of spiritual aura readings and my meditation practice, refined my consciousness quite beautifully. I felt the light of the Soul present within my life and shared much love, healing and joy with friends, students and family.

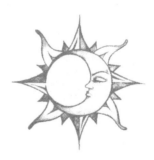